HEALTH AND HUMAN DEVELOPMENT

CLINICAL ONCOLOGY

AN ENCOMPASSING OVERVIEW

HEALTH AND HUMAN DEVELOPMENT

JOAV MERRICK - SERIES EDITOR

NATIONAL INSTITUTE OF CHILD HEALTH
AND HUMAN DEVELOPMENT,
MINISTRY OF SOCIAL AFFAIRS, JERUSALEM

Clinical Oncology: An Encompassing Overview
Joav Merrick, Ariel Tenenbaum, Victoria Rico and Carlo DeAngelis (Editors)
2020. ISBN: 978-1-53617-933-0 (Hardcover)
2020. ISBN. 978-1-53617-934-7 (eBook)

Pain: Perspectives on Acute and Chronic Pain
Patricia Schofield, Ariel Tenenbaum, Joav Merrick (Editors)
2020: ISBN: 978-1-53617-748-0 (Hardcover)
2020: ISBN: 978-1-53617-749-7 (eBook)

Animal-Assisted Interventions for Health and Human Service Professionals
Carlie J. Driscoll
2020. ISBN: 978-1-53617-433-5 (Hardcover)
2020. ISBN: 978-1-53617-434-2 (eBook)

Cancer Management in Latin America II: Melanoma to Cost-Effectiveness
Maurício F Silva, Gustavo Nader Marta, Luis CM Antunes, Fiona Lim, Bo Angela Wan, Beatriz Amendola, Joav Merrick (Editors)
2020. ISBN: 978-1-53616-735-1 (Hardcover)
2020. ISBN: 978-1-53616-736-8 (eBook)

Cancer Management in Latin America I: Nasopharyngeal to Renal Cancer
Maurício F Silva, Gustavo Nader Marta, Luis CM Antunes, Fiona Lim, Bo Angela Wan, Beatriz Amendola, Joav Merrick (Editors)
2020. ISBN: 978-1-53616-733-7 (Hardcover)
2020. ISBN: 978-1-53616-734-4 (eBook)

Alternative Medicine Research Yearbook 2017
Joav Merrick (Editor)
2018. ISBN: 978-1-53613-726-2 (Hardcover)
2018. ISBN: 978-1-53613-727-9 (eBook)

Clinical Art Psychotherapy with War Veterans
Alexander Kopytin and Alexey Lebedev
2018. ISBN: 978-1-53612-975-5 (Softcover)
2017. ISBN: 978-1-53612-976-2 (eBook)

Cancer and Exercise
Leila Malek, Fiona Lim, Bo Angela Wan, Patrick L Diaz, Edward Chow, Joav Merrick (Editors)
2018. ISBN: 978-1-53612-747-8 (Hardcover)
2018. ISBN: 978-1-53612-748-5 (eBook)

Brennan Healing Science: An Integrative Approach to Therapeutic Intervention
Nina Koren, Muriel Moreno and Joav Merrick (Editors)
2018. ISBN: 978-1-53612-825-3 (Hardcover)
2018. ISBN: 978-1-53612-826-0 (eBook)

Palliative Care: Oncology Experience from Hong Kong
Louisa Cheuk-Yu Lui, Kam-Hung Wong, Rebecca Yeung, Joav Merrick (Editors)
2017. ISBN: 978-1-53612-397-5 (Softcover)
2017. ISBN: 978-1-53612-430-9 (eBook)

Psychosocial Needs: Success in Life and Career Planning
Daniel TL Shek, Janet TY Leung, Tak Y Lee and Joav Merrick (Editors)
2017. ISBN: 978-1-53611-951-0 (Hardcover)
2017. ISBN: 978-1-53611-971-8 (eBook)

Cannabis: Medical Aspects
Blair Henry, Arnav Agarwal, Edward Chow, Hatim A Omar, and Joav Merrick (Editors)
2017. ISBN: 978-1-53610-510-0 (Hardcover)
2017. ISBN: 978-1-53610-522-3 (eBook)

Palliative Care: Psychosocial and Ethical Considerations
Blair Henry, Arnav Agarwal, Edward Chow, and Joav Merrick (Editors)
2017. ISBN: 978-1-53610-607-7 (Hardcover)
2017. ISBN: 978-1-53610-611-4 (eBook)

Oncology: The Promising Future of Biomarkers
Anthony Furfari, George S Charames, Rachel McDonald, Leigha Rowbottom, Azar Azad, Stephanie Chan, Bo Angela Wan, Ronald Chow, Carlo DeAngelis, Pearl Zaki, Edward Chow and Joav Merrick (Editors)
2017. ISBN: 978-1-53610-608-4 (Hardcover)
2017. ISBN: 978-1-53610-610-7 (eBook)

Public Health Yearbook 2016
Joav Merrick (Editor)
2017. ISBN: 978-1-53610-947-4 (Hardcover)
2017. ISBN: 978-1-53610-956-6 (eBook)

Alternative Medicine Research Yearbook 2016
Joav Merrick (Editor)
2017. ISBN: 978-1-53610-972-6 (Hardcover)
2017. ISBN: 978-1-53611-000-5 (eBook)

Pain Management Yearbook 2016
Joav Merrick (Editor)
2017. ISBN: 978-1-53610-949-8 (Hardcover)
2017. ISBN: 978-1-53610-959-7 (eBook)

Medical Cannabis: Clinical Practice
Shannon O'Hearn, Alexia Blake, Bo Angela Wan, Stephanie Chan, Edward Chow and Joav Merrick (Editors)
2017. ISBN: 978-1-53611-907-7 (Softcover)
2017. ISBN: 978-1-53611-927-5 (eBook)

Cancer: Treatment, Decision Making and Quality of Life
Breanne Lechner, Ronald Chow, Natalie Pulenzas, Marko Popovic, Na Zhang, Xiaojing Zhang, Edward Chow, and Joav Merrick (Editors)
2016. ISBN: 978-1-63483-863-4 (Hardcover)
2015. ISBN: 978-1-63483-882-5 (eBook)

Cancer: Bone Metastases, CNS Metastases and Pathological Fractures
Breanne Lechner, Ronald Chow, Natalie Pulenzas, Marko Popovic, Na Zhang, Xiaojing Zhang, Edward Chow, and Joav Merrick (Editors)
2016. ISBN: 978-1-63483-949-5 (Hardcover)
2015. ISBN: 978-1-63483-960-0 (eBook)

Cancer: Spinal Cord, Lung, Breast, Cervical, Prostate, Head and Neck Cancer
Breanne Lechner, Ronald Chow, Natalie Pulenzas, Marko Popovic, Na Zhang, Xiaojing Zhang, Edward Chow and Joav Merrick (Editors)
2016. ISBN: 978-1-63483-904-4 (Hardcover)
2015. ISBN: 978-1-63483-911-2 (eBook)

Cancer: Survival, Quality of Life and Ethical Implications
Breanne Lechner, Ronald Chow, Natalie Pulenzas, Marko Popovic, Na Zhang, Xiaojing Zhang, Edward Chow and Joav Merrick (Editors)
2016. ISBN: 978-1-63483-905-1 (Hardcover)
2015. ISBN: 978-1-63483-912-9 (eBook)

Cancer: Pain and Symptom Management
Breanne Lechner, Ronald Chow, Natalie Pulenzas, Marko Popovic, Na Zhang, Xiaojing Zhang, Edward Chow, and Joav Merrick (Editors)
2016. ISBN: 978-1-63483-905-1 (Hardcover)
2015. ISBN: 978-1-63483-881-8 (eBook)

Alternative Medicine Research Yearbook 2015
Joav Merrick (Editor)
2016. ISBN: 978-1-63484-511-3 (Hardcover)
2016. ISBN: 978-1-63484-542-7 (eBook)

Public Health Yearbook 2015
Joav Merrick (Editor)
2016. ISBN: 978-1-63484-511-3 (Hardcover)
2016. ISBN: 978-1-63484-546-5 (eBook)

Quality, Mobility and Globalization in the Higher Education System: A Comparative Look at the Challenges of Academic Teaching
Nitza Davidovitch, Zehavit Gross, Yuri Ribakov, and Anna Slobodianiuk (Editors)
2016. ISBN: 978-1-63484-986-9 (Hardcover)
2016. ISBN: 978-1-63485-012-4 (eBook)

Alternative Medicine Research Yearbook 2014
Joav Merrick (Editor)
2015. ISBN: 978-1-63482-161-2 (Hardcover)
2015. ISBN: 978-1-63482-205-3 (eBook)

Pain Management Yearbook 2014
Joav Merrick (Editor)
2015. ISBN: 978-1-63482-164-3 (Hardcover)
2015. ISBN: 978-1-63482-208-4 (eBook)

Public Health Yearbook 2014
Joav Merrick (Editor)
2015. ISBN: 978-1-63482-165-0 (Hardcover)
2015. ISBN: 978-1-63482-209-1 (eBook)

Forensic Psychiatry: A Public Health Perspective
Leo Sher and Joav Merrick (Editors)
2015. ISBN: 978-1-63483-339-4 (Hardcover)
2015. ISBN: 978-1-63483-346-2 (eBook)

Leadership and Service Learning Education: Holistic Development for Chinese University Students
Daniel TL Shek, Florence KY Wu and Joav Merrick (Editors)
2015. ISBN: 978-1-63483-340-0 (Hardcover)
2015. ISBN: 978-1-63483-347-9 (eBook)

Mental and Holistic Health: Some International Perspectives
Joseph L Calles Jr, Donald E Greydanus, and Joav Merrick (Editors)
2015. ISBN: 978-1-63483-589-3 (Hardcover)
2015. ISBN: 978-1-63483-608-1 (eBook)

India: Health and Human Development Aspects
Joav Merrick (Editor)
2014. ISBN: 978-1-62948-784-7 (Hardcover)
2014. ISBN: 978-1-62948-794-6 (eBook)

Alternative Medicine Research Yearbook 2013
Joav Merrick (Editor)
2014. ISBN: 978-1-63321-094-3 (Hardcover)
2014. ISBN: 978-1-63321-144-5 (eBook)

Health Consequences of Human Central Obesity
Kaushik Bose and Raja Chakraborty (Editors)
2014. ISBN: 978-1-63321-152-0 (Hardcover)
2014. ISBN: 978-1-63321-181-0 (eBook)

Public Health Yearbook 2013
Joav Merrick (Editor)
2014. ISBN: 978-1-63321-095-0 (Hardcover)
2014. ISBN: 978-1-63321-097-4 (eBook)

Public Health: Improving Health via Inter-Professional Collaborations
Rosemary M Caron and Joav Merrick (Editors)
2014. ISBN: 978-1-63321-569-6 (Hardcover)
2014. ISBN: 978-1-63321-594-8 (eBook)

Textbook on Evidence-Based Holistic Mind-Body Medicine: Holistic Practice of Traditional Hippocratic Medicine
Søren Ventegodt and Joav Merrick
2013. ISBN: 978-1-62257-105-5 (Hardcover)
2012. ISBN: 978-1-62257-174-1 (eBook)

Textbook on Evidence-Based Holistic Mind-Body Medicine: Healing the Mind in Traditional Hippocratic Medicine
Søren Ventegodt and Joav Merrick
2013. ISBN: 978-1-62257-112-3 (Hardcover)
2012. ISBN: 978-1-62257-175-8 (eBook)

Textbook on Evidence-Based Holistic Mind-Body Medicine: Sexology and Traditional Hippocratic Medicine
Søren Ventegodt and Joav Merrick
2013. ISBN: 978-1-62257-130-7 (Hardcover)
2012. ISBN: 978-1-62257-176-5 (eBook)

Health and Happiness from Meaningful Work: Research in Quality of Working Life
Søren Ventegodt and Joav Merrick (Editors)
2013. ISBN: 978-1-60692-820-2 (Hardcover)
2009. ISBN: 978-1-61324-981-9 (eBook)

Conceptualizing Behavior in Health and Social Research: A Practical Guide to Data Analysis
Said Shahtahmasebi and Damon Berridge
2013. ISBN: 978-1-60876-383-2 (Hardcover)
2013. ISBN: 978-1-53611-212-2 (eBook)

Adolescence and Sports
Dilip R Patel, Donald E Greydanus, Hatim Omar and Joav Merrick (Editors)
2013. ISBN: 978-1-60876-702-1 (Hardcover)
2010. ISBN: 978-1-61761-483-5 (eBook)

Pediatric and Adolescent Sexuality and Gynecology: Principles for the Primary Care Clinician
Hatim A Omar, Donald E Greydanus, Artemis K. Tsitsika, Dilip R. Patel and Joav Merrick (Editors)
2013. ISBN: 978-1-60876-735-9 (Softcover)

Human Development: Biology from a Holistic Point of View
Søren Ventegodt, Tyge Dahl Hermansen and Joav Merrick
2013. ISBN: 978-1-61470-441-6 (Hardcover)
2011. ISBN: 978-1-61470-541-3 (eBook)

Building Community Capacity: Case Examples from Around the World
Rosemary M Caron and Joav Merrick (Editors)
2013. ISBN: 978-1-62417-175-8 (Hardcover)
2013. ISBN: 978-1-62417-176-5 (eBook)

Managed Care in a Public Setting
Richard Evan Steele
2013. ISBN: 978-1-62417-970-9 (Softcover)
2013. ISBN: 978-1-62417-863-4 (eBook)

Bullying: A Public Health Concern
Jorge C Srabstein and Joav Merrick (Editors)
2013. ISBN: 978-1-62618-564-7 (Hardcover)
2013. ISBN: 978-1-62618-588-3 (eBook)

Bedouin Health: Perspectives from Israel
Joav Merrick, Alean Al-Krenami and Salman Elbedour (Editors)
2013. ISBN: 978-1-62948-271-2 (Hardcover)
2013: ISBN: 978-1-62948-274-3 (eBook)

Health Promotion: Community Singing as a Vehicle to Promote Health
Jing Sun, Nicholas Buys and Joav Merrick (Editors)
2013. ISBN: 978-1-62618-908-9 (Hardcover)
2013: ISBN: 978-1-62808-006-3 (eBook)

Public Health Yearbook 2012
Joav Merrick (Editor)
2013. ISBN: 978-1-62808-078-0 (Hardcover)
2013: ISBN: 978-1-62808-079-7 (eBook)

Alternative Medicine Research Yearbook 2012
Joav Merrick (Editor)
2013. ISBN: 978-1-62808-080-3 (Hardcover)
2013: ISBN: 978-1-62808-079-7 (eBook)

Advanced Cancer: Managing Symptoms and Quality of Life
Natalie Pulenzas, Breanne Lechner, Nemica Thavarajah, Edward Chow, and Joav Merrick (Editors)
2013. ISBN: 978-1-62808-239-5 (Hardcover)
2013: ISBN: 978-1-62808-267-8 (eBook)

Treatment and Recovery of Eating Disorders
Daniel Stein and Yael Latzer (Editors)
2013. ISBN: 978-1-62808-248-7 (Softcover)

Health Promotion: Strengthening Positive Health and Preventing Disease
Jing Sun, Nicholas Buys and Joav Merrick (Editors)
2013. ISBN: 978-1-62257-870-2 (Hardcover)
2013: ISBN: 978-1-62808-621-8 (eBook)

Pain Management Yearbook 2011
Joav Merrick (Editor)
2013. ISBN: 978-1-62808-970-7 (Hardcover)
2013: ISBN: 978-1-62808-971-4 (eBook)

Pain Management Yearbook 2012
Joav Merrick (Editor)
2013. ISBN: 978-1-62808-973-8 (Hardcover)
2013: ISBN: 978-1-62808-974-5 (eBook)

Suicide from a Public Health Perspective
Said Shahtahmasebi and Joav Merrick
2013. ISBN: 978-1-62948-536-2 (Hardcover)
2014: ISBN: 978-1-62948-537-9 (eBook)

Food, Nutrition and Eating Behavior
Joav Merrick and Sigal Israeli (Editors)
2013. ISBN: 978-1-62948-233-0 (Hardcover)
2013: ISBN: 978-1-62948-234-7 (eBook)

Public Health Concern: Smoking, Alcohol and Substance Use
Joav Merrick and Ariel Tenenbaum (Editors)
2013. ISBN: 978-1-62948-424-2 (Hardcover)
2013. ISBN: 978-1-62948-430-3 (eBook)

Mental Health from an International Perspective
Joav Merrick, Shoshana Aspler and Mohammed Morad (Editors)
2013. ISBN: 978-1-62948-519-5 (Hardcover)
2013. ISBN: 978-1-62948-520-1 (eBook)

Adolescence and Chronic Illness. A Public Health Concern
Hatim Omar, Donald E Greydanus, Dilip R Patel and Joav Merrick (Editors)
2012. ISBN: 978-1-60876-628-4 (Hardcover)
2010. ISBN: 978-1-61761-482-8 (eBook)

Child and Adolescent Health Yearbook 2009
Joav Merrick (Editor)
2012. ISBN: 978-1-61668-913-1 (Hardcover)
2012. ISBN: 978-1-62257-095-9 (eBook)

Child and Adolescent Health Yearbook 2010
Joav Merrick (Editor)
2012. ISBN: 978-1-61209-788-6 (Hardcover)
2012. ISBN: 978-1-62417-046-1 (eBook)

Child Health and Human Development Yearbook 2010
Joav Merrick (Editor)
2012. ISBN: 978-1-61209-789-3 (Hardcover)
2012. ISBN: 978-1-62081-721-6 (eBook)

Public Health Yearbook 2010
Joav Merrick (Editor)
2012. ISBN: 978-1-61209-971-2 (Hardcover)
2012. ISBN: 978-1-62417-863-4 (eBook)

Alternative Medicine Yearbook 2010
Joav Merrick (Editor)
2012. ISBN: 978-1-62100-132-4 (Hardcover)
2011. ISBN: 978-1-62100-210-9 (eBook)

The Astonishing Brain and Holistic Consciousness: Neuroscience and Vedanta Perspectives
Vinod D Deshmukh
2012. ISBN: 978-1-61324-295-7

Health Risk Communication
Marijke Lemal and Joav Merrick (Editors)
2012. ISBN: 978-1-62257-544-2 (Hardcover)
2012. ISBN: 978-1-62257-552-7 (eBook)

Translational Research for Primary Healthcare
Erica Bell, Gert P Westert and Joav Merrick (Editors)
2012. ISBN: 978-1-61324-647-4 (Hardcover)
2012. ISBN: 978-1-62417-409-4 (eBook)

Our Search for Meaning in Life: Quality of Life Philosophy
Søren Ventegodt and Joav Merrick
2012. ISBN: 978-1-61470-494-2 (Hardcover)
2011. ISBN: 978-1-61470-519-2 (eBook)

Randomized Clinical Trials and Placebo: Can You Trust the Drugs are Working and Safe?
Søren Ventegodt and Joav Merrick
2012. ISBN: 978-1-61470-067-8 (Hardcover)
2011. ISBN: 978-1-61470-151-4 (eBook)

Building Community Capacity: Minority and Immigrant Populations
Rosemary M Caron and Joav Merrick (Editors)
2012. ISBN: 978-1-62081-022-4 (Hardcover)
2012. ISBN: 978-1-62081-032-3 (eBook)

Applied Public Health: Examining Multifaceted Social or Ecological Problems and Child Maltreatment
John R Lutzker and Joav Merrick (Editors)
2012. ISBN: 978-1-62081-356-0 (Hardcover)
2012. ISBN: 978-1-62081-388-1 (eBook)

Treatment and Recovery of Eating Disorders
Daniel Stein and Yael Latzer (Editors)
2012. ISBN: 978-1-61470-259-7 (Hardcover)
2012. ISBN: 978-1-61470-418-8 (eBook)

Human Immunodeficiency Virus (HIV) Research: Social Science Aspects
Hugh Klein and Joav Merrick (Editors)
2012. ISBN: 978-1-62081-293-8 (Hardcover)
2012. ISBN: 978-1-62081-346-1 (eBook)

AIDS and Tuberculosis: Public Health Aspects
Daniel Chemtob and Joav Merrick (Editors)
2012. ISBN: 978-1-62081-382-9 (Softcover)
2012. ISBN: 978-1-62081-406-2 (eBook)

Public Health Yearbook 2011
Joav Merrick (Editor)
2012. ISBN: 978-1-62081-433-8 (Hardcover)
2012. ISBN: 978-1-62081-434-5 (eBook)

Alternative Medicine Research Yearbook 2011
Joav Merrick (Editor)
2012. ISBN: 978-1-62081-476-5 (Hardcover)
2012. ISBN: 978-1-62081-477-2 (eBook)

Building Community Capacity: Skills and Principles
Rosemary M Caron and Joav Merrick (Editors)
2012. ISBN: 978-1-61209-331-4 (Hardcover)
2012. ISBN: 978-1-62257-238-0 (eBook)

Textbook on Evidence-Based Holistic Mind-Body Medicine: Basic Principles of Healing in Traditional Hippocratic Medicine
Søren Ventegodt and Joav Merrick
2012. ISBN: 978-1-62257-094-2 (Hardcover)
2012. ISBN: 978-1-62257-172-7 (eBook)

Textbook on Evidence-Based Holistic Mind-Body Medicine: Basic Philosophy and Ethics of Traditional Hippocratic Medicine
Søren Ventegodt and Joav Merrick
2012. ISBN: 978-1-62257-052-2 (Hardcover)
2013. ISBN: 978-1-62257-707-1 (eBook)

Textbook on Evidence-Based Holistic Mind-Body Medicine: Research, Philosophy, Economy and Politics of Traditional Hippocratic Medicine
Søren Ventegodt and Joav Merrick
2012. ISBN: 978-1-62257-140-6 (Hardcover)
2012. ISBN: 978-1-62257-171-0 (eBook)

Behavioral Pediatrics, 3rd Edition
Donald E Greydanus, Dilip R Patel, Helen D Pratt and Joseph L Calles, Jr (Editors)
2011. ISBN: 978-1-60692-702-1 (Hardcover)
2009. ISBN: 978-1-60876-630-7 (eBook)

Rural Child Health: International Aspects
Erica Bell and Joav Merrick (Editors)
2011. ISBN: 978-1-60876-357-3 (Hardcover)
2011. ISBN: 978-1-61324-005-2 (eBook)

International Aspects of Child Abuse and Neglect
Howard Dubowitz and Joav Merrick (Editors)
2011. ISBN: 978-1-60876-703-8 (Hardcover)
2010. ISBN: 978-1-61122-049-0 (Softcover)
2010. ISBN: 978-1-61122-403-0 (eBook)

Environment, Mood Disorders and Suicide
Teodor T Postolache and Joav Merrick (Editors)
2011. ISBN: 978-1-61668-505-8 (Hardcover)
2011. ISBN: 978-1-62618-340-7 (eBook)

Positive Youth Development: Evaluation and Future Directions in a Chinese Context
Daniel TL Shek, Hing Keung Ma and Joav Merrick (Editors)
2011. ISBN: 978-1-60876-830-1 (Hardcover)
2011. ISBN: 978-1-62100-175-1 (Softcover)
2010. ISBN: 978-1-61209-091-7 (eBook)

Understanding Eating Disorders: Integrating Culture, Psychology and Biology
Yael Latzer, Joav Merrick and Daniel Stein (Editors)
2011. ISBN: 978-1-61728-298-0 (Hardcover)
2011. ISBN: 978-1-61470-976-3 (Softcover)
2011. ISBN: 978-1-61942-054-0 (eBook)

Advanced Cancer Pain and Quality of Life
Edward Chow and Joav Merrick (Editors)
2011. ISBN: 978-1-61668-207-1 (Hardcover)
2010. ISBN: 978-1-61668-400-6 (eBook)

Positive Youth Development: Implementation of a Youth Program in a Chinese Context
Daniel TL Shek, Hing Keung Ma and Joav Merrick (Editors)
2011. ISBN: 978-1-61668-230-9

Social and Cultural Psychiatry Experience from the Caribbean Region
Hari D Maharajh and Joav Merrick (Editors)
2011. ISBN: 978-1-61668-506-5 (Hardcover)
2010. ISBN: 978-1-61728-088-7 (eBook)

Narratives and Meanings of Migration
Julia Mirsky
2011. ISBN: 978-1-61761-103-2 (Hardcover)
2010. ISBN: 978-1-61761-519-1 (eBook)

Self-Management and the Health Care Consumer
Peter William Harvey
2011. ISBN: 978-1-61761-796-6 (Hardcover)
2011. ISBN: 978-1-61122-214-2 (eBook)

Sexology from a Holistic Point of View
Soren Ventegodt and Joav Merrick
2011. ISBN: 978-1-61761-859-8 (Hardcover)
2011. ISBN: 978-1-61122-262-3 (eBook)

Principles of Holistic Psychiatry: A Textbook on Holistic Medicine for Mental Disorders
Soren Ventegodt and Joav Merrick
2011. ISBN: 978-1-61761-940-3 (Hardcover)
2011. ISBN: 978-1-61122-263-0 (eBook)

Clinical Aspects of Psychopharmacology in Childhood and Adolescence
Donald E Greydanus, Joseph L Calles, Jr, Dilip P Patel, Ahsan Nazeer and Joav Merrick (Editors)
2011. ISBN: 978-1-61122-135-0 (Hardcover)
2011. ISBN: 978-1-61122-715-4 (eBook)

Climate Change and Rural Child Health
Erica Bell, Bastian M Seidel and Joav Merrick (Editors)
2011. ISBN: 978-1-61122-640-9 (Hardcover)
2011. ISBN: 978-1-61209-014-6 (eBook)

Rural Medical Education: Practical Strategies
Erica Bell, Craig Zimitat and Joav Merrick (Editors)
2011. ISBN: 978-1-61122-649-2 (Hardcover)
2011. ISBN: 978-1-61209-476-2 (eBook)

Advances in Environmental Health Effects of Toxigenic Mold and Mycotoxins
Ebere Cyril Anyanwu
2011. ISBN: 978-1-60741-953-2
2011. ISBN: 978-1-53611-209-2

Public Health Yearbook 2009
Joav Merrick (Editor)
2011. ISBN: 978-1-61668-911-7 (Hardcover)
2011. ISBN: 978-1-62417-365-3 (eBook)

Child Health and Human Development Yearbook 2009
Joav Merrick (Editor)
2011. ISBN: 978-1-61668-912-4

Alternative Medicine Yearbook 2009
Joav Merrick (Editor)
2011. ISBN: 978-1-61668-910-0 (Hardcover)
2011. ISBN: 978-1-62081-710-0 (eBook)

The Dance of Sleeping and Eating among Adolescents: Normal and Pathological Perspectives
Yael Latzer and Orna Tzischinsky (Editors)
2011. ISBN: 978-1-61209-710-7 (Hardcover)
2011. ISBN: 978-1-62417-366-0 (eBook)

Drug Abuse in Hong Kong: Development and Evaluation of a Prevention Program
Daniel TL Shek, Rachel CF Sun and Joav Merrick (Editors)
2011. ISBN: 978-1-61324-491-3 (Hardcover)
2011. ISBN: 978-1-62257-232-8 (eBook)

Chance Action and Therapy: The Playful Way of Changing
Uri Wernik
2010. ISBN: 978-1-60876-393-1 (Hardcover)
2011. ISBN: 978-1-61122-987-5 (Softcover)
2011. ISBN: 978-1-61209-874-6 (eBook)

Bone and Brain Metastases: Advances in Research and Treatment
Arjun Sahgal, Edward Chow and Joav Merrick (Editors)
2010. ISBN: 978-1-61668-365-8 (Hardcover)
2010. ISBN: 978-1-61728-085-6 (eBook)

Challenges in Adolescent Health: An Australian Perspective
David Bennett, Susan Towns, Elizabeth Elliott and Joav Merrick (Editors)
2009. ISBN: 978-1-60741-616-6 (Hardcover)
2009. ISBN: 978-1-61668-240-8 (eBook)

Obesity and Adolescence: A Public Health Concern
Hatim A Omar, Donald E Greydanus, Dilip R Patel and Joav Merrick (Editors)
2009. ISBN: 978-1-60692-821-9 (Hardcover)
2009. ISBN: 978-1-61470-465-2 (eBook)

Poverty and Children: A Public Health Concern
Alexis Lieberman and Joav Merrick (Editors)
2009. ISBN: 978-1-60741-140-6 (Hardcover)
2009. ISBN: 978-1-61470-601-4 (eBook)

Living on the Edge: The Mythical, Spiritual, and Philosophical Roots of Social Marginality
Joseph Goodbread
2009. ISBN: 978-1-60741-162-8 (Hardcover)
2013. ISBN: 978-1-61122-986-8 (Softcover)
2011. ISBN: 978-1-61470-192-7 (eBook)

Alcohol-Related Cognitive Disorders: Research and Clinical Perspectives
Leo Sher, Isack Kandel and Joav Merrick (Editors)
2009. ISBN: 978-1-60741-730-9 (Hardcover)
2009. ISBN: 978-1-60876-623-9 (eBook)

Children and Pain
Patricia Schofield and Joav Merrick (Editors)
2009. ISBN: 978-1-60876-020-6 (Hardcover)
2009. ISBN: 978-1-61728-183-9 (eBook)

Complementary Medicine Systems: Comparison and Integration
Karl W Kratky
2008. ISBN: 978-1-60456-475-4 (Hardcover)
2008. ISBN: 978-1-61122-433-7 (eBook)

Pain in Children and Youth
Patricia Schofield and Joav Merrick (Editors)
2008. ISBN: 978-1-60456-951-3 (Hardcover)
2008. ISBN: 978-1-61470-496-6 (eBook)

Adolescent Behavior Research: International Perspectives
Joav Merrick and Hatim A Omar (Editors)
2007. ISBN: 1-60021-649-8

HEALTH AND HUMAN DEVELOPMENT

CLINICAL ONCOLOGY

AN ENCOMPASSING OVERVIEW

ARIEL TENENBAUM, MD
VICTORIA RICO
CARLO DEANGELIS
AND
JOAV MERRICK, MD, MMEDSCI, DMSC
EDITORS

nova
Medicine & Health
New York

Library of Congress Cataloging-in-Publication Data

Names: Tenenbaum, Ariel, editor. | Rico, Victoria, editor. | DeAngelis, Carlo, editor. | Merrick, Joav, 1950- editor.
Title: Clinical oncology : an encompassing overview / Ariel Tenenbaum, Victoria Rico, Carlo DeAngelis, Joav Merrick, editors. Description: New York : Nova Science Publishers, [2020] | Series: Health and human development | Includes bibliographical references and index. | Summary: "In this book we have gathered recent research related to cancer and cancer treatment and care. We also present research on pharmacy in cancer treatment, a few papers on breast cancer, research on bone metastases, radiation therapy and some pilot programs on telemedicine in cancer care, prostate cancer screening in Guyana, cost analysis of metastatic non-small cell lung cancer in Canada and early oncology rehabilitation for lymphoma patients in Singapore. We hope this research will be of interest to our readers"-- Provided by publisher.
Identifiers: LCCN 2020018362 (print) | LCCN 2020018363 (ebook) | ISBN 9781536179330 (paperback) | ISBN 9781536179347 (adobe pdf) Subjects: LCSH: Cancer--Treatment. | Oncology.
Classification: LCC RC270.8 .C546 2020 (print) | LCC RC270.8 (ebook) | DDC 616.99/4--dc23
LC record available at https://lccn.loc.gov/2020018362
LC ebook record available at https://lccn.loc.gov/2020018363

Published by Nova Science Publishers, Inc. † New York

CONTENTS

INTRODUCTION

In: Clinical Oncology
Editors: Ariel Tenenbaum et al.
ISBN: 978-1-53617-933-0

Chapter 1

ONCOLOGY PHARMACIST EXPERTISE IN CANCER CARE

Victoria Rico[1,*], Carlo DeAngelis[1], PharmD, Ariel Tenenbaum[2-4], MD and Joav Merrick[3-6], MD, MMedSci, DMSc

[1]Sunnybrook Odette Cancer Centre, University of Toronto, Toronto, Ontario, Canada
[2]Center for Children with Chronic Diseases and Down Syndrome Center Jerusalem, Jerusalem, Israel
[3]Department of Pediatrics, Mt Scopus Campus, Hadassah Hebrew University Medical Center, Jerusalem, Israel
[4]National Institute of Child Health and Human Development, Jerusalem, Israel
[5]Kentucky Children's Hospital, University of Kentucky, Lexington, Kentucky, United States of America
[6]Center for Healthy Development, School of Public Health, Georgia State University, Atlanta, Georgia, United States of America

* Corresponding Author's Email: Edward.Chow@sunnybrook.ca.

ABSTRACT

Oncology pharmacy is a specialty within pharmacy practice that involves general pharmacy knowledge and skills, coupled with expertise in cancer treatment and management. An increasing number of oncology pharmacists are becoming involved in assisting with direct patient care, decision making and education, and in some settings, are providing direct patient care themselves. Utilizing the knowledge and expertise of oncology pharmacists in cancer care settings, such as through basic counselling, or through the implementation of pharmacy callback programs, can improve patient knowledge and education, patient quality of life, and patient treatment outcomes. In this book we have gathered recent research related to cancer and cancer treatment and care. We also present research on pharmacy in cancer treatment, a few papers on breast cancer, research on bone metastases, radiation therapy and some pilot programs on telemedicine in cancer care, prostate cancer screening in Guyana, cost analysis of metastatic non-small cell lung cancer in Canada and early oncology rehabilitation for lymphoma patients in Singapore. We hope this research will be of interest to our readers.

INTRODUCTION

Oncology pharmacists play an important role in optimizing the quality of care that is provided to patients undergoing cancer treatment. Oncology pharmacy is a specialty within pharmacy practice that involves general pharmacy knowledge and skills, coupled with expertise in cancer treatment and management. An increasing number of oncology pharmacists are becoming involved in assisting with direct patient care, decision making and education, and in some settings, are providing direct patient care themselves (1).

A systematic literature review identified articles that discussed the value and utility of oncology pharmacists in healthcare settings, and across the available literature found that oncology pharmacists play a valuable role in four main areas, including clinical care, patient education, informatics and technology, and economic savings (2). Several studies have documented pharmacist led interventions that contributed to health outcomes of patients, to the management of patient care, and to documentation in electronic medical records (3–5). For example, Muluneh et al. (6) evaluated a pharmacy guided oral chemotherapy management program, and among other factors, examined medication adherence rates, pharmacy provided interventions, and molecular response rates among patients with chronic myeloid leukemia (6). This study found that the pharmacy-led program resulted in enhanced knowledge of oral chemotherapy among patients, improved oral chemotherapy adherence rates, and improved major molecular response rates relative to the molecular response rates of patients with chronic myeloid leukemia documented in the literature (6).

A randomized controlled study assessed the efficacy of pharmaceutical care and interventions on chemotherapy knowledge-attitude-practice, and quality of life amongst patients receiving treatment for cancer (7). This study found that upon completion of the study, the patients in the pharmaceutical intervention group (who received comprehensive pharmaceutical care and written medication information) had significantly increased scores in both the knowledge-attitude-practice dimension and the quality of life dimension, while there was no difference observed in the attitude, practice, and quality of life scores amongst the control group (7). The findings of this study suggest that pharmacy teams can positively influence patient knowledge on chemotherapy, improve their ability to address adverse reactions to chemotherapy, and enhance their quality of life during cancer treatment (7).

Another study examined a telephone call back program for antibiotic therapy that was established to reinforce pharmacy counseling and to monitor patients' progress throughout antibiotic therapy (8). Telephone call backs were made to 521 patients, and it was found that 47 of the 79 patients that experienced unsuccessful antibiotic treatment repeated the first treatment or began a new antibiotic regimen without visiting a physician. This study concluded that implementing a pharmacy callback program can be a cost-effective and clinically valuable method to monitor and enhance therapeutic drug outcomes in patients (8).

Several studies and programs have documented the value that oncology pharmacists have in the care and treatment outcomes of patients undergoing cancer therapies. Thus, utilizing the knowledge and expertise of oncology pharmacists in cancer care settings, such as through basic counselling, or through the implementation of pharmacy callback programs, can improve patient knowledge and education, patient quality of life, and patient treatment outcomes.

REFERENCES

[1] Sessions JK, Valgus J, Barbour SY, Iacovelli L. Role of Oncology Clinical Pharmacists in Light of the Oncology Workforce Study. J Oncol Pract 2010;6(5):270–2.

[2] M Segal E, Bates J, Fleszar SL, Holle LM, Kennerly-Shah J, Rockey M, et al. Demonstrating the value of the oncology pharmacist within the healthcare team. J Oncol Pharm Pract 2019;25(8):1945–67.

[3] Ruder AD, Smith DL, Madsen MT, Kass FH. Is there a benefit to having a clinical oncology pharmacist on staff at a community oncology clinic? J Oncol Pharm Pract 2011;17(4):425–32.

[4] Patel JM, Holle LM, Clement JM, Bunz T, Niemann C, Chamberlin KW. Impact of a pharmacist-led oral chemotherapy-monitoring program in patients with metastatic castrate-resistant prostate cancer. J Oncol Pharm Pract 2016;22(6):777–83.

[5] McNamara E, Redoutney L, Mackler E, Severeson J, Petersen L, Mahmood T. Improving Oral Oncolytic Patient Self-Management. J Oncol Pract 2016;12(9):e864–9.

[6] Muluneh B, Schneider M, Faso A, Amerine L, Daniels R, Crisp B, et al. Improved adherence rates and clinical outcomes of an integrated, closed-loop, pharmacist-led oral chemotherapy management program. J Oncol Pract 2018;14(6):e324–34.

[7] Wang Y, Wu H, Xu F. Impact of clinical pharmacy services on KAP and QOL in cancer patients: A single-center experience. Biomed Res Int 2015;2015:1–8.

[8] Westfall GR, Narducci WA. A community-pharmacy-based callback program for antibiotic therapy. J Am Pharm Assoc (Wash) 1997;NS37(3):330–4.

SECTION ONE: PHARMACY IN ONCOLOGY

In: Clinical Oncology
Editors: Ariel Tenenbaum et al.
ISBN: 978-1-53617-933-0

Chapter 2

REVIEW OF A PHARMACIST-LED TELEPHONE FOLLOW-UP PROGRAM FOR AMBULATORY PATIENTS RECEIVING CHEMOTHERAPY AT A TERTIARY CANCER CENTRE

Carmilia Sun, PharmD, Ronald Chow,
Philomena Sousa, MBA, Carlo DeAngelis, PharmD,
Flay Charbonneau, Stephanie Chan,
and Mark Pasetka*, PharmD
Odette Cancer Centre, Sunnybrook Health Sciences Centre,
University of Toronto, Toronto, Canada

ABSTRACT

The Odette Cancer Centre (OCC) Pharmacy's clinical call-back program provides teaching and advice for patients new to receiving chemotherapy. Trained pharmacists and pharmacy students initiate and facilitate calls to

* Corresponding Author's E-mail: mark.pasetka@sunnybrook.ca.

follow-up with patients at home one to three days after their first treatment. During these calls the pharmacist/student assesses and manages patients with respect to presence and severity of treatment-related toxicities. The aim of this chapter was to describe a pharmacist-led telephone follow-up program in patients receiving parenteral anticancer therapy at the OCC through a retrospective chart review. From June 2013 to June 2016, 6,984 calls were made, of which 5,511 (78.9%) successfully reached patients. 3,184 unique patients were called, and the percentage of patients requiring more calls in the latter years declined. While the total proportion of successful calls fell year-after-year, the number of patients who were never reached declined, highlighting the positive reception of this program. Future studies should investigate patient satisfaction, information learned, actions taken as a result of the follow-ups, and clinical outcomes.

INTRODUCTION

Intravenous antineoplastic agents have been extensively used for decades to treat various types of cancer; however, models of care in cancer centres across Canada have not been standardized. Prior to patients receiving their first session of chemotherapy, they are educated on the process and effects of their specific chemotherapy regimen. On the day of chemotherapy administration, patients usually have blood work and vital signs assessed by a nurse or oncologist, after which, if deemed to be acceptable, they proceed to receive pre-medications and chemotherapy. Patients are then discharged home the same day and often with a follow-up appointment booked to see their oncologist in clinic prior to the second cycle of chemotherapy. The monitoring of patients once at home is often absent, leaving the onus on patients to call-in if treatment-related toxicities (TRTs) arise, which leads to a reactive-style of patient care in comparison to proactively contacting and assessing patients in order to mitigate side effects before they become significant.

Antineoplastics typically possess a narrow therapeutic index and many have a high-risk for toxicity which requires appropriate preventative management, often in the form of pharmaceutical agents; however, the utilization of supportive care medications may require patient-specific tailoring by a healthcare professional (1). In centres that do not proactively assess patients for TRTs, these modifications may occur too late or not until the next treatment or appointment with their oncologist. Therefore, it is imperative that patients be mindful of common adverse effects associated with their regimen, ways to prevent them, and strategies to manage them if and/or when they occur. Patients also need to be made aware of any drug-drug, drug-disease, and drug-nutrient interactions prior to pursuing treatment or starting any new supportive medications. As pharmaceutical experts and key members of the interdisciplinary team, oncology pharmacists are in an ideal position to provide pre-treatment education and follow-up for patients receiving chemotherapy (2). Several studies have demonstrated the value of clinical oncology pharmacists in teaching and proactive follow-up for patients on chemotherapy treatment (3-5).

It is believed that pharmacy clinical services are an essential part of the centre's provision of patient-centred care; thus, it is important to understand the scope of the current program and identify areas for improvement. In addition, to our knowledge there have not been any studies assessing the number of patients reached via a pharmacy-led chemotherapy call-back program; therefore, this information could aid in better defining standards for clinical oncology pharmacy practice. The aim of this study was to assess the breadth and workload of the pharmacist-led telephone follow-up program in patients receiving parenteral anticancer therapy at the Odette Cancer Centre (OCC) in Toronto, Canada.

OUR STUDY

The duties of OCC pharmacy are divided between fulfilling the centre's medication dispensing needs (parenteral/oral chemotherapy and supportive medications) and participating in direct patient care (or what was historically referred to as "cognitive services") (5). These include patient education, treatment monitoring/follow-up, toxicity management, and communication with other medical professionals.

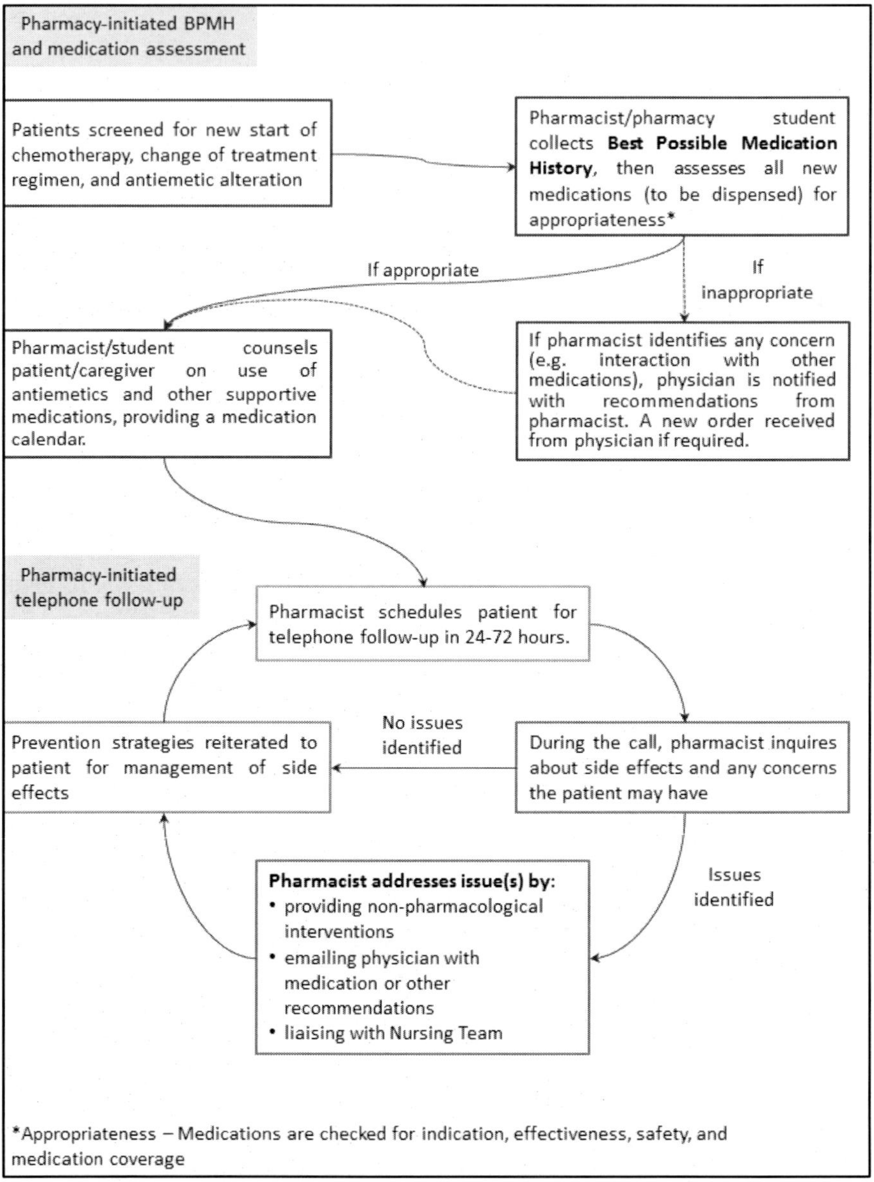

Figure 1. Odette cancer centre pharmacy chemotherapy suite workflow outline.

Since its inception, the pharmacy call-back program has provided teaching and advice to patients who have received traditional intravenous chemotherapy and targeted agents. Any patient who is starting a new treatment regimen, restarting a prior regimen (following a break from therapy), or those who have had changes made to their supportive medications receive counseling and therapeutic follow-up. Trained pharmacists and pharmacy students initiate and facilitate calls to follow-up with patients at home 24 to 72 hours after their first treatment, restart, or supportive care alteration. During these calls the pharmacist/student assesses patients for chemotherapy-induced toxicities, such as chemotherapy-induced nausea and vomiting (CINV), constipation, diarrhoea, mucositis, and other treatment-specific toxicities such as neuropathy and ototoxicity; supportive care interventions are provided to help patients manage medication-related issues (see Figure 1). Pharmacists or students would then document and communicate with the rest of the oncology team to provide suggestions for medication management and future follow up. It currently requires 4-5 pharmacy students in addition to 1-3 pharmacists on a daily basis to maintain the service. Considering the telephone follow-up rosters were recorded on paper up until early June 2013, only electronic data (recorded in Excel spreadsheets) was analyzed from that point onward.

Design and study population

This was a retrospective study, whereby chart review was conducted to determine the number of patients called by the Odette Cancer Centre Pharmacy from June 5, 2013 to June 30, 2016. Patients were identified using the centre's computerized physician order entry system, OPIS (Oncology Patient Information System), and chemotherapy scheduling system, CHARM (Chemotherapy Appointment Reservation Manager). This retrospective review was approved by Sunnybrook Health Sciences Centre's research ethics board. All patients who received parenteral antineoplastics as an outpatient at the OCC between June 5, 2013 and June 30, 2016 were included in the call-back program if any of the following criteria were met:

1. Patient receiving first chemotherapy treatment with two or more supportive medications.
2. Patient receiving a new treatment regimen (i.e., received different chemotherapy regimen in the past) with two or more supportive medications.
3. Patient had changes made to supportive medication(s) based on adverse effects experienced after previous cycle(s).
4. Patient has not received treatment in three or more months.

Patients on certain clinical trial treatments may have been excluded as they had standard protocols and adverse effect management guidelines to follow. Identification of patients enrolled in the follow-up program was done through the follow-up roster (spreadsheet) maintained in the OCC Pharmacy as part of the program. Only patients with complete information recorded on the roster were included in this review.

Program characterization

In order to characterize the program, the following information was gathered and separated by year:

1. Total number of follow-up calls made
2. Number of unique patients reached
3. Number of patients reached on first, second, and subsequent attempts
4. Number of patients never reached and most common reasons why (if recorded)
5. Number of patients who required more than one follow-up call (i.e., issues were identified and follow-up on was performed based on recommendations made).

Data analysis

Data was documented and compiled in Microsoft Excel® worksheets, and descriptive statistics (e.g., mean, median, percentage) were used to report the desired outcomes. Percentages were calculated based on the total number of patients called for follow-up and grouped by year.

FINDINGS

Table 1. Patient characteristics

Variable		*n*	(%)
Age (years)			
Median	61		
Range	13-92		
Gender			
Male		1346	(43.4%)
Female		1758	(56.6%)
Treatment Intent			
Neoadjuvant		653	(21.0%)
Adjuvant		971	(31.3%)
Curative		320	(10.3%)
Palliative		1160	(37.4%)
Primary Cancer Site			
Gastrointestinal		761	(24.5%)
Gynaecological		690	(22.2%)
Lymphoma		369	(11.9%)
Lung		340	(11.0%)
Head & Neck		331	(10.7%)
Breast		175	(5.6%)
Genitourinary		165	(5.3%)
Leukemia		54	(1.7%)
Multiple myeloma		53	(1.7%)
Skin		50	(1.6%)
Other/unknown		118	(3.8%)

Between June 5, 2013 and June 30, 2016, a total of 6984 calls were made from the OCC Pharmacy, Broken down by year, 1316 were made in 2013, 2228 in 2014, 2424 in 2015, and 1005 in 2016. Of those calls, 5511

(78.9%) were successful in connecting with the patient/caregiver for telephone follow-up. These were termed "successful call attempts". The percentage of successful call attempts has been declining year after year: 93.8% in 2013, 85.6% in 2014, 72.6% in 2015, and 60.6% in 2016 (thus far) (see Table 1).

Table 2. Outcomes of interest to assess feasibility of OCC pharmacy's call-back program

Outcome	Year				Overall
	2013	**2014**	**2015**	**2016**	**2013-2016**
Total Attempts	1316	2228	2424	1005	6984
Total Successfully Reached	1235 (93.8%)	1908 (85.6%)	1759 (72.6%)	609 (60.6%)	5511 (78.9%)
No. of Unique Patients	726	1022	1000	436	3184
No. of Patients Never Reached	102 (14.0%)	88 (8.6%)	91 (9.1%)	33 (7.6%)	314 (9.9%)
No. of Patients Requiring:					
1 Call	726 (100%)	1022 (100%)	1000 (100%)	436 (100%)	3184 (100%)
2 Calls	403 (55.5%)	565 (55.3%)	541 (54.1%)	213 (48.9%)	1722 (54.1%)
3 Calls	230 (31.7%)	317 (31.0%)	301 (30.1%)	83 (19.0%)	931 (29.2%)
4 Calls	108 (14.9%)	177 (17.3%)	172 (17.2%)	28 (6.4%)	485 (15.2%)
5 Calls	65 (9.0%)	102 (10.0%)	94 (9.4%)	12 (2.8%)	372 (8.6%)
>5 Calls	83 (11.4%)	180 (17.6%)	128 (12.8%)	5 (1.1%)	396 (12.4%)
No. of Patients Successfully Reached After:					
1 Call	556 (76.6%)	835 (81.7%)	796 (79.6%)	342 (78.4%)	2529 (79.4%)
2 Calls	59 (8.1%)	81 (7.9%)	92 (9.2%)	51 (11.7%)	283 (8.9%)
3 Calls	9 (1.2%)	13 (1.3%)	21 (2.1%)	10 (2.3%)	53 (1.7%)
4 Calls	1 (0.1%)	4 (0.4%)	2 (0.2%)	0 (0%)	7 (0.2%)
5 Calls	1 (0.1%)	1 (0.1%)	1 (0.1%)	0 (0%)	3 (0.1%)
>5 Calls	0 (0%)	0 (0%)	0 (0%)	0 (0%)	0 (0%)

OCC Pharmacy called 726, 1022, 1759, and 436 unique patients in 2013, 2014, 2015, and 2016 respectively, summing 3943 patients over the investigative period. A total of 314 patients (9.9%) were never reached, with the two most commonly cited reasons being a busy line and patients feeling unwell thus not wanting to talk. Patients not reached over the years amounted to 14%, 8.6%, 9.1%, and 7.6% each year from 2013 to 2016, respectively (see Table 2).

All patients who met the criteria received a first call from OCC Pharmacy. However, a total of 1722 (54.1%) patients warranted a second call (55.5% in 2013, 55.3% in 2014, 54.1% in 2015, 48.9% in 2016), 931 (29.2%) patients required a third call (31.7% in 2013, 31.0% in 2014, 30.1% in 2015, 19.0% in 2016), and expectedly decreasing percentages received subsequent follow-up calls (see Figure 2). Two patients received 14 calls, one patient received 13 calls, and two patients received 12 calls.

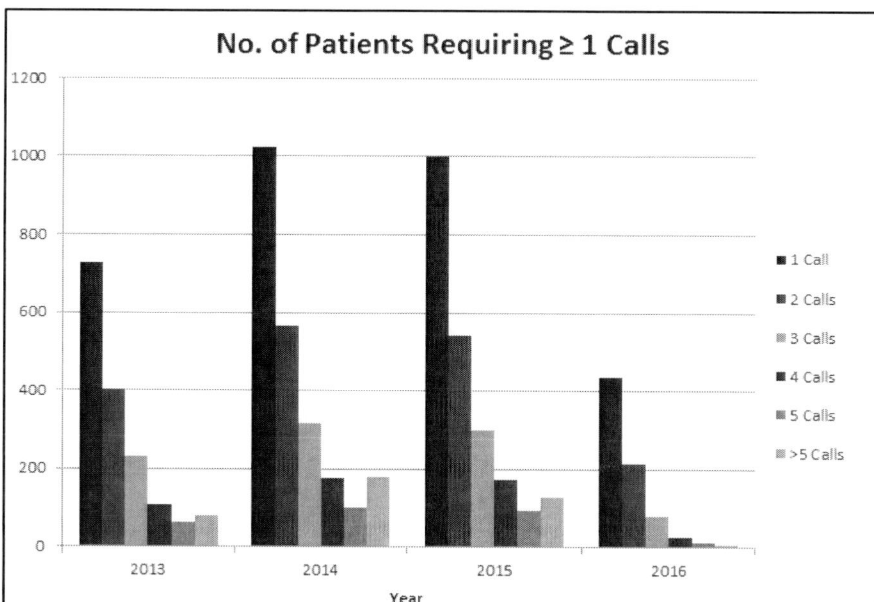

Figure 2. Number of patients requiring ≥ 1 follow-up calls from our program broken down by year.

In 2013, 556 (76.6%) patients were reached at the first call. The following years, 835 (81.7%), 796 (79.6%), and 342 (78.4%) were successfully reached at the first call in 2014, 2015, and 2016 respectfully. A total of 283 (8.9%) patients required two calls to be reached – 59 (8.1%) in 2013, 81 (7.9%) in 2014, 92 (9.2%) in 2015, and 51 (11.7%) in 2016. The number of patients reached after three calls added up to 53 (1.7%) with 9 (1.2%) in 2013, 13 (1.3%) in 2014, 21 (2.1%) in 2015, and 10 (2.3%) in 2016. Finally, there were seven (0.2%) patients who were called four times and three (0.1%) who were called five times in order to be reached once (see Figure 3).

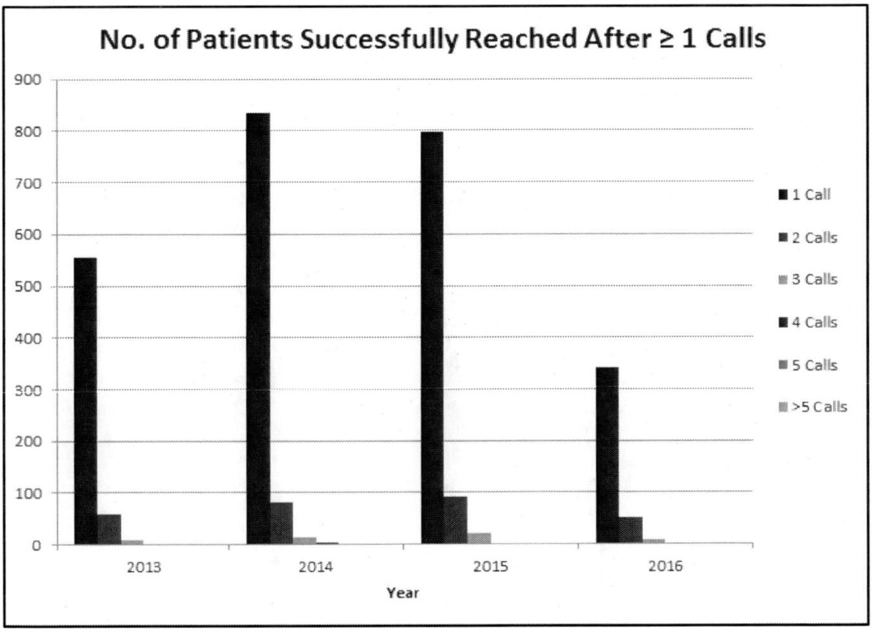

Figure 3. Number of patients reached after *n* calls each year.

Discussion

This is the first study to assess the number of patients reached via a pharmacy-led chemotherapy call-back program, and documents a highly-utilized program. In viewing the results, note that statistics for the year of 2013 began on June 5, and those for the year of 2016 ended on June 30. Thus, it is difficult to comment on trends in the number of patients reached versus number of calls made as these years were not fully investigated. While the percentage of successful interactions ("successful call attempts") after one call seems to have declined over the years, it may not actually have decreased as the data has not accounted for the months from July to December of year 2016. The percentage of patients reached for follow-up after two or three calls has increased over the years, and the proportion of patients never reached declined. With this trend, it would appear that the Odette Cancer Centre Pharmacy is making more calls to reach a similar number of patients as years go by. However, this may not necessarily affect feasibility of the program as unsuccessful attempts at contacting patients do not require much time on the phone. Moreover, fewer additional/subsequent follow-up calls were made as years went by, likely decreasing the amount of time spent following up on recommendations made. This is by no means indicative of the efficacy or inefficacy of pharmacy interventions.

This study demonstrates that the practice of regular telephone follow-up by a pharmacist and student team is achievable. More in-depth feasibility analyses should be performed by collecting data on time spent with patients on the phone (recorded beginning in 2015) and the number of pharmacy staff (pharmacists and students) involved per day. This will help determine whether the program is feasible all year-round, including several weeks where there may be a shortage of pharmacy students. With further analysis of these data, future studies should match patients according to baseline characteristics; identify commonly reported adverse events, pharmacist recommendations, number of communications sent to oncologists or nursing teams; and investigate the results of all pharmacy-made interventions. Patient satisfaction and ease of understanding should also be examined as studies performed in other centres have had promising results in these aspects (3-5). This could best be performed prospectively with surveys, but preliminary data can be obtained retrospectively based on follow-up conversations and outcomes. Additionally, the degree of provider satisfaction in the program should also be assessed and include aspects of student confidence in providing recommendations, improvement in efficiency, and acquisition of clinical skills.

A study done at the Princess Margaret Cancer Centre in Toronto, Canada, evaluated the patient-perceived impact of clinical pharmacy services and proactive follow-up care in an ambulatory chemotherapy unit (3). Results showed that 95.5% of patients (n = 112) found the time spent with a pharmacist at the initial chemotherapy session was worthwhile, and 92.9% of patients answered "Yes, absolutely" to meeting with a pharmacist at the start of chemotherapy being important. Interactions with a pharmacist increased patients' understanding of their medication regimens 92.6% of the time (n = 108). Furthermore, follow-up calls were considered worthwhile by 92.6% of patients (n = 82), and 86% of patients (n = 93) were "very satisfied" or "satisfied" with the service. Pharmacists also had the ability to help patients manage adverse effects at home for 91.4% of the time (n = 93) (3). Another study performed at a cancer centre in the United States (Texas) had similar outcomes with 86.4% of patients stating it was "absolutely necessary" to meet with a pharmacist and 74% stating that they understood how to take their medications after speaking with a pharmacist (4).

Likewise, a study done in China assessed quality of life (QOL) and chemotherapy knowledge-attitude-practice (KAP) in patients receiving pharmaceutical intervention compared to standard medical care. A questionnaire (KAP questionnaire) was administered to all patients, assessing their knowledge of chemotherapy, its associated side effects, and management (i.e., when to go to ER); attitude toward chemotherapy and its adverse effects; and practice/behaviour (i.e., assessing alcohol use and mindsets on medical advice). The pharmaceutical intervention group received an information booklet outlining the purpose of chemotherapy, how to prepare for treatment and the assessments involved, strategies for prevention and management of adverse drug reactions, and cautions for oral chemotherapy drugs. Patients in this group also received face-to-face medication education and psychological counseling services with a clinical pharmacist twice per week for two months. As might be expected, results showed that patients who received the pharmaceutical intervention had significantly greater KAP and QOL scores ($p < 0.05$). Additionally, nausea/vomiting, pain, sleep disturbance, constipation, and diarrhea were significantly reduced in the intervention group ($p < 0.05$) (5).

All three prior studies demonstrated the value of clinical oncology pharmacists in teaching and proactive follow-up for patients on chemotherapy treatment (3-5). Coupled with our study, which demonstrates the workability of a follow-up program run by pharmacists and pharmacy students, pharmacists should be involved in patient education and monitoring at more tertiary institutions across the country.

This study was not without limitations. The records had instances where data was not complete – busy pharmacists may have called patients for follow-up but, with many other tasks at hand, were unable to document the interaction. This situation led to a proportion of patients who unfortunately could not be reviewed, as it was not possible to determine whether a follow-up had been conducted or not. Additionally, statistical analyses were not conducted to determine whether observed trends (decreases and increases) were significantly different as this was not necessary to assess the program.

It is difficult to comment on the program's feasibility in this study as time analyses and number of staff/students required to perform follow-up tasks were not examined. While it does not quantitatively or qualitatively document patient satisfaction as do prior studies (3-4), it does show a program that has successfully carried out its objective of connecting with patients to provide pharmaceutical and supportive care.

Overall, this pharmacist-initiated telephone follow-up program appears to be achievable and has great potential. Anecdotally, it seems to be well-received by patients and reaching its objective of providing routine and ongoing supportive care. Further investigations should look into patient satisfaction, patient learning, and actions taken due to follow-up calls, as well as the subsequent outcomes.

Results indicate that a relatively consistent percentage of ambulatory patients receiving parenteral antineoplastics have been called by the Odette Cancer Centre Pharmacy each year from 2013 to 2016. With each passing year, fewer patients are being missed (unable to contact for follow-up) and fewer additional follow-up calls are being required.

These results do not prove the effectiveness of the program, but do show that it has been conductible for a long period of time since its inception in year 2000. Based on the results of this study and the known value of oncology pharmacy clinical services, further investigations should be performed to determine time spent with patients, patient satisfaction and understanding, as well as commonly reported adverse effects and results of recommended management strategies, amongst others.

ACKNOWLEDGMENTS

We would like to acknowledge and thank all the University of Waterloo School of Pharmacy and University of Toronto School of Pharmacy students, as well as all pharmacy residents and fellows who provided clinical care in this program.

REFERENCES

[1] Jaehde U, Liekweg A, Simons S, Westfeld M. Minimising treatment-associated risks in systemic cancer therapy. Pharm World Sci 2008;30(2):161-8.

[2] Holle LM and Boehnke Michaud L. Oncology pharmacists in health care delivery: vital members of the cancer care team. J Oncol Pract 2014;10(3):e142-5.

[3] Crespo A and Tyszka M. Evaluating the patient-perceived impact of clinical pharmacy services and proactive follow-up care in an ambulatory chemotherapy unit. J Oncol Pharm Pract 2017;23(4). doi: 10.1177/1078155216634180.

[4] McKee M, Frei BL, Garcia A, Fike D, Soefje SA. Impact of clinical pharmacy services on patients in an outpatient chemotherapy academic clinic. J Oncol Pharm Pract 2011;17(4):387-94.

[5] Wang Y, Wu H and Xu F. Impact of clinical pharmacy services on KAP and QOL in cancer patients: a single-centre experience. Biomed Res Int 2015;2015:502431.

In: Clinical Oncology
Editors: Ariel Tenenbaum et al.
ISBN: 978-1-53617-933-0

Chapter 3

About the Pharmacy Call-Back Program at the Odette Cancer Centre, Sunnybrook Health Sciences Centre, Toronto, Canada

Victoria Rico*[*] *and Carlo DeAngelis, PharmD
Sunnybrook Odette Cancer Centre, University of Toronto,
Toronto, Ontario, Canada

Abstract

At the Odette Cancer Centre at Sunnybrook Health Sciences Centre in Toronto, Ontario, Canada a telephone call-back program is offered where pharmacists and pharmacy students provide education and advice to patients who recently began chemotherapy treatment. These phone calls take place one to three days following a patient's first cycle of chemotherapy, and during these calls the pharmacist or pharmacy students assess chemotherapy related toxicities or side effects. In cases where patients are experiencing toxicities, the pharmacy team helps to

[*] Corresponding Author's E-mail: victoria.g.rico@hotmail.com.

manage these toxicities by implementing an intervention over the telephone.

INTRODUCTION

The Odette Cancer Centre at Sunnybrook Health Sciences Centre in Toronto, Ontario, Canada offers a telephone call-back program where pharmacists and pharmacy students provide education and advice to patients who recently began chemotherapy treatment (1). These phone calls take place one to three days following a patient's first cycle of chemotherapy, and during these calls the pharmacist or pharmacy students assess chemotherapy related toxicities or side effects (1). In cases where patients are experiencing toxicities, the pharmacy team helps to manage these toxicities by following up over the telephone and implementing an intervention (2). Such interventions can range from suggesting the use of a baking soda rinse for mucositis, to altering anti-emetic regimens due to severe chemotherapy induced nausea and vomiting.

A retrospective chart review of patients receiving parenteral anticancer therapy at the Odette Cancer Centre was conducted by Sun et al. to investigate the scope of the pharmacy-led callback program at this centre (1). This review found that 6,984 phone calls were made between June 2013 and June 2016, and 5,511 (78.9%) of these phone calls were successful in contacting the patient (1). Further, this study found that the proportion of patients who were unsuccessfully contacted by the pharmacy declined over the years (1). Such results demonstrate that since the Odette Cancer Centre's initiation of this call-back program in the year 2000, it has been feasible for a long period of time and has been positively received by those involved in it (1).

Another retrospective chart review was conducted by Rico et al. to evaluate the efficacy of pharmacy led interventions conducted over the telephone in patients receiving adjuvant or neoadjuvant chemotherapy for breast cancer at the Odette Cancer Centre from 2010 to 2015 (2). In this study, 1,666 pharmacy led interventions that were implemented for 444 patients with breast cancer were analyzed. Side effects addressed by these interventions included nausea, vomiting, constipation, diarrhea, mucositis, and others. Due to this study's retrospective nature, a high proportion of the outcomes of the interventions were undocumented or immeasurable. However, of those that had documented success, approximately 84% were successful, while approximately 15% were unsuccessful. As such, this demonstrates that pharmacy interventions provided over the telephone to patients undergoing chemotherapy treatment can reduce side-effects experienced by patients (2).

REFERENCES

[1] Sun C, Chow R, Sousa P, DeAngelis C, Charbonneau F, Chan S, et al. Review of a pharmacist-led telephone follow-up program for ambulatory patients receiving chemotherapy at a tertiary cancer centre. J Pain Manag 2018;11(2):171–9.

[2] Rico V, Lao M, Goodall S, Asthana R, Wang K, D'Souza R, et al. Impact of pharmacy interventions in patients receiving chemotherapy for breast cancer at the Odette Cancer Centre. J Oncol Pharm Pract 2019;25(5):14.

SECTION TWO: BREAST CANCER

In: Clinical Oncology
Editors: Ariel Tenenbaum et al.
ISBN: 978-1-53617-933-0

Chapter 4

RADIATION-INDUCED MORPHEA OF THE BREAST FIVE YEARS POST-TREATMENT: A CASE REPORT

Emily Lam, Caitlin Yee, Leah Drost, Gina Wong, Erin McKenzie, Edward Chow, and Danny Vesprini*, MD

Odette Cancer Centre, Sunnybrook Health Sciences Centre,
University of Toronto, Toronto, Ontario, Canada

ABSTRACT

Radiation-induced morphea is a rare but well-documented skin reaction that presents months to years after radiation therapy. Occurring most frequently in patients receiving radiotherapy for breast cancer, it is often misdiagnosed as recurrent cancer and presents a challenging treatment

* Corresponding Author: Danny Vesprini, MD, MSc, FRCPC Department of Radiation Oncology, Odette Cancer Centre, Sunnybrook Health Sciences Centre, 2075 Bayview Avenue, Toronto ON, Canada. E-mail: danny.vesprini@sunnybrook.ca.

plan for clinicians, as there is no known cause and the efficacy of various treatment options is disputed. We report the case of a 69-year-old woman who presented with post-irradiation morphea approximately five years after radiation treatment. To our knowledge, this is the sixth reported case of radiation-induced morphea occurring outside of the radiation field in a breast cancer patient. The patient was treated with topical steroids and methotrexate injections which did not clear the rash but allowed for better management of the condition. Due to the limited availability of similar cases reported in the literature, the treatment and outcomes for patients with radiation-induced morphea are not well-understood and require further research.

INTRODUCTION

Radiation-induced morphea (RIM), also known as localized scleroderma, is a rare, fibrosing disorder of the dermis and/or subcutaneous tissues (1, 2). Characterized by indurated papular lesions, erythematous plaques and pigmentary changes, RIM is frequently misdiagno 28, 2019.sed as metastatic carcinoma or recurrent disease (3, 4). Mild skin reactions following radiotherapy (RT) of the breast are common, appearing in approximately 90% of breast cancer patients (5). These reactions generally heal without serious intervention approximately 2 to 4 weeks after RT has ended (6, 7). In contrast, RIM is a painful and disfiguring condition which can occur months to years after RT, and affects approximately 0.2% of breast cancer patients receiving RT (3). RIM typically occurs in two clinical phases: phase one is marked by pain and edema, and phase two, referred to as burnout, occurs months after phase one and presents as changes in pigmentation, induration and fibrosis of the skin (2).

We present the case of a 69-year-old woman with RIM following treatment for a triple-negative, left-sided invasive ductal carcinoma (IDC).

CASE STORY

In 2011, a 62-year-old woman was diagnosed with a grade III, triple negative, left-sided IDC with no lymphovascular invasion following mammogram and ultrasound core biopsy.

The patient underwent a lumpectomy and sentinel lymph node biopsy. The closest surgical margin was 1 cm, and both sentinel lymph nodes removed were negative for malignancy. She recovered well from the surgery and was scheduled for four cycles of taxotere and cyclophosphamide.

During her first cycle of chemotherapy, the patient developed an erythematous rash with a severe burning sensation on the dorsal surface of her hands, abdomen and external vaginal area. She was prescribed a topical steroid cream which did not resolve the issue.

Following her last cycle of chemotherapy, the patient began adjuvant radiation of 50 Gray (Gy) in 25 fractions with a simultaneous integrated boost of 13.25 Gy in 25 fractions to the surgical bed. Upon completion of RT, the patient experienced very mild patches of erythema on the medial aspect of her treated left breast.

Approximately five years after her initial diagnosis of IDC, the patient presented with a painful circumferential rash with central clearing on her left breast. The rash was eczematous and mildly pruritic, and progressed over approximately three to four months.

Magnetic resonance imaging of the breast ruled out sclerosing metastatic breast adenocarcinoma. Four biopsies of the rash showed resemblance to inflammatory morphea and the patient was prescribed fluocinonide cream for approximately two months. The cream was ineffective in clearing the rash: pain persisted, tingling sensations appeared and morphea began spreading to the upper left back and right arm. Physical examination revealed RIM with ulcerated lichen sclerosis overlap, characterized by white indurated plaques with several areas of red soft plaques covering the left breast.

The patient also developed lichen sclerosis on her bilateral arms and upper thighs approximately eight months after her initial diagnosis of RIM.

The lichen sclerosis continued to worsen over two months, spreading to her vulva and perineum with ulcerating features. The patient was prescribed Lamisil and 1% hydrocortisone cream which she reported greatly improved the pruritus and burning sensation in her genital area.

The patient was prescribed 20mg methotrexate (MTX) injections once weekly and 5mg folic acid daily. Although the patient tolerated the injections well, the rash continued to fluctuate and spread across the left breast. At the patient's three-month follow-up, three areas of erosion surrounding the RIM were reported and the weekly dose of MTX was increased to 25mg by her dermatologist. The patient reported slight improvements to the lesions 7 months after receiving the initial MTX injection and after 9 months the RIM was well-controlled.

After two years of MTX without any side effects, the patient's RIM showed moderate improvement. The patient reported ongoing irritation of the plaque located under her left breast and was given a 2.5mg/mL intralesional steroid injection (2cc total), which made the pain more manageable. At last follow-up, approximately two years after initial MTX treatment, the patient's RIM was stable while receiving a weaning dose of 17.5 mg MTX injections.

DISCUSSION

Due to its rarity, treatments for RIM have historically been unsatisfactory; a review of 54 reported cases since 1989 has reported insufficient treatment options (8). The causes of RIM are unclear, and although in some cases RIM resolves spontaneously, a majority of patients report minimal or no improvements despite intensive treatment (9, 10). Additionally, there is no apparent relation between the dose of radiation and RIM (11).

Early biopsies can be useful to rule out other skin complications, guide subsequent management and minimize patient morbidity (12). Diagnoses based on exclusion are most commonly utilized for RIM; after ruling out cellulitis or inflammatory breast cancer recurrence, dermatologists may begin treatments targeted for RIM (12).

The patient described in this report developed inflammatory morphea approximately five years post-RT, which is later than the average onset for RIM, typically reported around 3 years post-RT (9). The patient did experience several common skin reactions in the weeks following RT, such as erythema and dry desquamation. However, following treatment there was no indication of unusual skin reactions during her follow-up appointments with her radiation oncologist.

A majority of reported RIM cases remain confined to the radiation field and surrounding tissues; however, approximately 20 to 25% of reported RIM cases describe distant skin involvement (13). The patient discussed in this report developed systemic signs which are uncommon among patients with RIM. Only five cases of breast cancer patients with RIM and distant skin involvement of the lower extremities and groin area have previously been reported in the literature (14–18). Similar to the case described by Ullén and Björkholm, our patient presented with lower extremity involvement approximately 6 years post-RT which is later than the average onset of the other three cases mentioned above. Based on the limited number of reported cases of RIM with lower extremity involvement in breast cancer patients, treatment options are not well-defined.

In a 24-week trial of low-dose oral MTX for nine individuals with widespread morphea, participants responded well to treatment and MTX decreased itchiness and tightness of the skin (19). In four retrospective studies published between 1997 and 2009, a total of 119 patients with morphea received a combination of MTX and systemic steroids resulting in a success rate of 79% according to clinician-reported skin quality (1). Echoing these results, the patient discussed in this report also reported moderate improvement to the skin following weekly injections of MTX.

Although the cause of RIM remains uncertain, its pathogenesis has been linked to the transforming growth factor-β (TGF-β). TGF-β inhibits the growth of endothelial cells and can strongly affect the stimulation of fibroblast synthesis (20). An increase in fibroblast activity has been linked to increase cytokine production which is believed to increase collagen synthesis (20). Accordingly, treatment options targeted at reducing cytokine production by decreasing collagen levels in the skin through Ultraviolet A (UVA) phototherapy have reported significant improvements in skin softening (21). While promising, the studies on UVA phototherapy for RIM have been limited by small sample sizes and this potential treatment option will require larger studies to better understand its utility.

CONCLUSION

This patient presented with inflammatory morphea five years after RT to the left breast. The patient received a common treatment of MTX and folic acid for morphea which moderately improved and stabilized the condition. Due to its rarity, the pathogenesis and treatment of RIM is not well-understood: therefore, more research is required to better understand optimal treatment and outcomes for patients with RIM and other late RT side effects.

ACKNOWLEDGMENTS

We thank the generous support of Bratty Family Fund, Michael and Karyn Goldstein Cancer Research Fund, Joey and Mary Furfari Cancer Research Fund, Pulenzas Cancer Research Fund, Joseph and Silvana Melara Cancer Research Fund, and Ofelia Cancer Research Fund.

REFERENCES

[1] Fett N, Werth VP. Update on morphea: Part II. Outcome measures and treatment. J Am Acad Dermatol 2011;64(2):231–42.

[2] Dyer BA, Hodges MG, Mayadev JS. Radiation-induced morphea: An under-recognized complication of breast irradiation. Clin Breast Cancer 2016;16(4):e141–3.

[3] Bleasel NR, Stapleton KM, Commens C, Ahern VA. Radiation-induced localized scleroderma in breast cancer patients. Australas J Dermatol 1999;40(2):99–102.

[4] Spalek M, Jonska-Gmyrek J, Gałecki J. Radiation-induced morphea - a literature review. J Eur Acad Dermatol Venereol 2015;29(2):197–202.

[5] Harper JL, Franklin LE, Jenrette JM, Aguero EG. Skin toxicity during breast irradiation: Pathophysiology and management. South Med J 2004;97(10):989–93.

[6] Salvo N, Barnes E, van Draanen J, Stacey E, Mitera G, Breen D, et al. Prophylaxis and management of acute radiation-induced skin reactions: a systematic review of the literature. Curr Oncol 2010;17(4):94–112.

[7] McQuestion M. Evidence-based skin care management in radiation therapy: Clinical update. Semin Oncol Nurs 2011;27(2):e1–17.

[8] Alhathlool A, Hein R, Andres C, Ring J, Eberlein B. Post-irradiation morphea: Case report and review of the literature. J Dermatol Case Rep 2012;6(3).

[9] Davis DA, Cohen PR, McNeese MD, Duvic M. Localized scleroderma in breast cancer patients treated with supervoltage external beam radiation: radiation port scleroderma. J Am Acad Dermatol 1996;35(6):923–7.

[10] Wernicke AG, Goltser Y, Trichter S, Sabbas A, Gaan J, Swistel AJ, et al. Introduction case report morphea as a consequence of accelerated partial breast irradiation. Clin Breast Cancer 2011;11(1):67–70.

[11] Colver GB, Rodger A, Mortimer PS, Savin JA, Neill SM, Hunter JA. Post-irradiation morphoea. Br J Dermatol 1989;120(6):831–5.

[12] Friedman O, Barnea Y, Hafner A. Underdiagnosed and disfiguring - Radiation-induced morphea following breast cancer treatment. Breast 2018;39:97-100.

[13] Fett N, Werth VP. Update on morphea Part I. Epidemiology, clinical presentation, and pathogenesis. J Am Acad Dermatol 2011;64:217–28.

[14] Ullen H, Björkholm E. Localized scleroderma in a woman irradiated at two sites for endometrial and breast carcinoma: a case history and a review of the literature. Int J Gynecol Cancer 2003;13(1):77-82.

[15] Akay BN, Sanli H, Heper AO. Postirradiation linear morphoea. Clin Exp Dermatol 2010;35(4):e106–8.

[16] Ardern-Jones MR, Black MM. Widespread morphoea following radiotherapy for carcinoma of the breast. Clin Exp Dermatol 2003;28(2):160–2.

[17] Kushi J, Csuka ME. Generalized morphea after breast cancer radiation therapy. Case Rep Rheumatol 2011;2011:951948.

[18] Yanaba K, Umezawa Y, Nakagawa H. A case of radiation-induced generalized morphea with prominent mucin deposition and tenderness. Am J Case Rep 2015;16:279–82.

[19] Seyger MMB, van den Hoogen FHJ, de Boo T, de Jong EMGJ. Low-dose methotrexate in the treatment of widespread morphea. J Am Acad Dermatol 1998;39(2):220–5.

[20] Smith EA, LeRoy EC. A possible role for transforming growth factor-β in systemic sclerosis. J Invest Dermatol 1990;95.

[21] El-Mofty M, Mostafa W, Esmat S, Youssef R, Bousseila M, Nagi N, et al. Suggested mechanisms of action of UVA phototherapy in morphea: a molecular study. Photodermatol Photoimmunol Photomed 2004;20(2):93–100.

In: Clinical Oncology
Editors: Ariel Tenenbaum et al.
ISBN: 978-1-53617-933-0

Chapter 5

ARE WE PROPERLY DIAGNOSING AND TREATING PAGET'S DISEASE OF THE BREAST? A CASE SERIES

Gina Wong, Leah Drost, Caitlin Yee, Emily Lam, Erin McKenzie, Heidi Gotthardt, Edward Chow and Danny Vesprini*, MD
Odette Cancer Centre, Sunnybrook Health Sciences Centre,
University of Toronto, Toronto, Ontario, Canada

ABSTRACT

Mammary Paget's disease (PD) is a rare occurrence that is highly associated with breast ductal carcinoma *in situ* (DCIS) and invasive ductal carcinoma (IDC). PD is characterized by aggressive changes to the nipple and areolar regions. Due to the rarity of this disease, evidence-based recommendations for management of PD are limited. Currently, mastectomy alone and breast conserving surgery paired with adjuvant

* Corresponding Author: Danny Vesprini MD, MSc, FRCPC. Department of Radiation Oncology, Odette Cancer Centre, Sunnybrook Health Sciences Centre, 2075 Bayview Avenue, Toronto, ON, Canada. E-mail: danny.vesprini@sunnybrook.ca.

radiation therapy (RT) are considered equally effective in treating PD. In this case series, two women presented with similar cases of PD of the nipple, though only one had associated DCIS; both women received or will receive RT after breast conserving surgery. PD is rare, and diagnosis is often missed or prolonged. More research on the treatment and outcomes of PD is recommended.

INTRODUCTION

Mammary Paget's disease (PD: also known as PD of the nipple) is a rare occurrence in breast cancer patients, associated with about 1 - 4% of all breast carcinomas (1). It presents more commonly in post-menopausal women aged 50-60 years, with a median age of 56 years (2).

Although this disease is uncommon, it does have a strong correlation with underlying breast cancer, as 92-100% of PD cases are associated with ductal carcinoma in situ (DCIS), invasive ductal carcinoma (IDC), or both (1, 3, 4).

PD involves the invasion of epidermal cells of the nipple and areola by malignant Paget's cells, often leading to excessive discolouration or pigmentation enclosed by an irregular border (1). The skin changes around the areola often cause discomfort and are generally described as thick, pigmented, moist, scaly and/or crusty, with extreme cases of ulceration (5). PD is often detected by an erythematous appearance and can be mistaken for chronic eczema or a rash, however the skin irritation associated with PD is more aggressive and persistent than a rash and diagnosis requires a skin punch biopsy to sample epithelial cells (6). Unlike common breast carcinomas where skin erythema is not an indicator of disease, PD skin abnormalities are a primary feature of disease (1, 6). Currently, there are no characteristics or features that have been identified as increasing the risk of PD (1).

This series presents two cases of PD, both with persistent areolar erythema. The first case is a 69-year-old woman diagnosed with PD and associated DCIS, and the second is a 64-year-old woman with PD and no associated underlying carcinoma.

CASE STORIES

Case 1

In late 2017, a 69-year-old woman presented with left nipple-areolar erythema, which had been present for approximately 3 years. She had clinician-reported ptosis of the breast, erythema and significant changes of the nipple bearing resemblance to an eczematous rash. She had no previous family history of breast or ovarian cancer and had no previous exposure to radiation.

A punch biopsy of her skin showed infiltration of the epidermis by atypical epithelioid cells and a high proportion of low molecular weight cytokines (CTK). The clinical and pathological findings led to diagnosis of PD. No palpable mass was detectable, and her initial mammogram was reported as normal. An MRI of her left breast found a lesion in her lower outer quadrant, and a subsequent biopsy revealed a benign tumour. However, due to the pathological diagnosis of PD, further investigation was indicated.

Due to the high correlation of breast cancer occurrence associated with mammary PD, the patient received central breast-conserving surgery (BCS) three months after the initial diagnosis. Final pathology revealed a 12mm grade 3 DCIS with no micro-invasion. There was no necrosis and her margins were widely negative (with the closest margin at 4 mm). Just over a month post-surgery, the patient received adjuvant radiotherapy (RT: 4256 centigray [cGy] in 16 fractions) to the left breast. Three months post RT, the patient returned for follow up and appeared to be recovering well, despite reporting mild hyperpigmentation and erythema. She agreed to return for annual follow-up appointments including mammograms and magnetic resonance imaging (MRI).

Case 2

In late 2018, a 64-year-old woman presented with a right-sided areolar rash which had persisted for 5 months. The rash contained small pustular-like lesions on the inferior aspect of her nipple, and the patient reported the skin surrounding her nipple to be quite raw, describing a tugging sensation with mild pruritus. After attempting multiple topical treatments, there was no change in her condition.

Mammogram and ultrasound were completed, and no underlying pathology or abnormality was detected. A week after initial presentation, a punch biopsy was completed revealing atypical cells with abundant pale cytoplasm within the epithelial cells; this confirmed a diagnosis of PD. One month after diagnosis, she returned with slight progression and mild scaling over her nipple, without palpable thickness.

Two months after the punch biopsy, an MRI of the right breast reported a lesion in the upper quadrant; however, a subsequent biopsy revealed a benign tumour. Two months after the biopsy, the patient received central BCS, of which final pathology revealed no associated DCIS or IDC. The patient is scheduled to receive 4256 cGy in 16 fractions to the right breast for the purpose of local control.

DISCUSSION

In both cases presented above, each patient's initial mammogram was normal, despite the presence of PD. Both patients presented with a benign tumour in the outer quadrants of their respective breasts. Patients with PD often do not have any palpable mass, making it difficult to identify IDC or DCIS clinically (6). Due to our incomplete understanding of the relationship between PD and malignancy, extensive imaging may be required to ensure diagnosis of potential underlying IDC or DCIS. In the cases reported above, neither patient had apparent associated malignancy through investigations, and it was only after the final pathology of the surgical specimen that the first patient was diagnosed with underlying

DCIS. A retrospective study by Sukumvanich et al. (7) reported that even in patients with no palpable mass, there was a higher likelihood of a high-grade carcinoma when PD was involved. In cases of PD with no other pathological findings, 27% of patients had associated IDC and 11% had sentinel lymph node involvement (7). The present case series echoes that in these types of cases, further investigation is warranted to rule out underlying malignancy; if not for the first patient's initial diagnosis of PD, her DCIS diagnosis would not have been identified. In contrast, the second patient had a similar experience to the first; however, after extensive imaging she did not appear to have any underlying DCIS or IDC. Although 92- 100% of all cases of PD are associated with DCIS or IDC (1,3,4), it is possible that this association is overestimated.

PD of the nipple is uncommon. However, the pathology of PD appears to be highly associated with underlying malignancy (1, 3, 4). PD cells act similarly to adenocarcinomas of the breast, as both tend to overexpress lower molecular weight CTK (1); this was seen in the first case. This link between carcinomas and PD cells with low molecular weight CTK may be the underlying cause of the malignant behaviour of PD, given that both of these cells share similar composition. The second case did report to have cells that were noticeably different than the epithelial cells, though the pathology did not comment on the expression of low molecular weight CTK. As reported above, the two cases had similar epithelial characteristics and composition, but one had underlying DCIS and the other had no underlying carcinoma. This could be a lead towards potential future research in the area of a PD, DCIS and CTK and would help increase our understanding of PD.

With regards to the management of PD, the most widely accepted practice is currently mastectomy (3,8,9). PD is essentially a typical case of breast carcinoma that is influenced by quickly growing Paget's cells; as in more typical carcinomas, there is potential utility for breast-conserving therapy in PD patients as well. A randomized controlled trial by Fisher et al. (10) found that in patients with IDC or DCIS, breast-conserving surgery with adjuvant RT had a low recurrence and re-irradiation rate similar to that of mastectomy. In PD patients, a meta-analysis by Li et al. (8) showed that the 5 year recurrence rate in patients who received mastectomy alone (5.6%) was not significantly different from patients treated with BCS and RT (6.6%). Similarly, in regards to PD of the nipple, Dixon et al. (11) reported that BCS coupled with adjuvant RT produced a similar recurrence to Li et al. of 6.0%. A study by Marshall et al. (12) further explored the efficacy of BCS+RT in PD patients, where they reported the 5 year local control rate to be 97%. In the second case, the patient did not have any DCIS present, however she agreed to proceed with RT to decrease the risk of PD recurrence or another malignant event. Although patients with PD have traditionally been offered mastectomy, the literature has shown that BCS+RT may be an effective alternative to reduce the risk of reoccurrence.

In both cases reported above, each patient received central BCS, to remove the affected epithelial cells and to prevent further spread of the Paget's cells. Both patients also received or are scheduled to receive postoperative RT, which is a recommended practice when paired with BCS (10). Wong et al. (9) found that only 50-55% of PD-IDC and PD-DCIS patients would receive BCS coupled with adjuvant RT, this number is quite low in terms of treatment usage and may suggest under treatment of a large group of patients. Some PD patients may feel as if they do not need further treatment after removal of the infected skin, but due to the association of PD and malignancy, post-operational RT is recommended (1, 9).

Although there is a high association between PD and underlying DCIS or IDC, one of the patients did not have underlying malignancy with her diagnosis of PD. This case series explores the idea that although there may be a strong association between PD and DCIS, more research is needed to understand this association. This case series also revealed that regardless of the presence of underlying disease, current treatment practices may be similar. Due to the ambiguity of the clinical and pathological features of this disease, more research is needed in this area to better guide optimal diagnosis and therapy.

Conclusion

PD diagnosis and its high association with underlying carcinoma place patients in a high-risk group and annual imaging is recommended. Mammary PD is easily overlooked, and diagnosis may be prolonged. The two cases presented above demonstrate that not all cases of PD have associated malignancy. So far, the most effective treatment for PD, mastectomy alone or BCS + adjuvant RT, is the same as that of typical breast carcinomas. However, due to the rarity of PD, more research is needed to identify and treat PD of the breast.

Acknowledgments

We thank the generous support of Bratty Family Fund, Michael and Karyn Goldstein Cancer Research Fund, Joey and Mary Furfari Cancer Research Fund, Pulenzas Cancer Research Fund, Joseph and Silvana Melara Cancer Research Fund, and Ofelia Cancer Research Fund.

References

[1] Karakas C. Paget's disease of the breast. J Carcinog 2011;10(1):31.

[2] Jamali FR, Ricci A, Deckers PJ. Paget's disease of the nipple-areola complex. Surg Clin North Am 1996;76(2):365–81.

[3] Wu Q, Ding X, Li J, Sun S, Zhu S, Wu J, et al. Surgical treatment in Paget's disease with invasive ductal carcinoma: an observational study based on SEER. Sci Rep 2017;7(1):45510.

[4] Amano G, Yajima M, Moroboshi Y, Kuriya Y, Ohuchi N. MRI accurately depicts underlying DCIS in a patient with Paget's disease of the breast without palpable mass and mammography findings. Jpn J Clin Oncol 2005;35(3):149–53.

[5] Paget J. On disease of the mammary areola preceding cancer of the mammary gland. CA Cancer J Clin 1971;21(5):303–4.

[6] Kothari AS, Beechey-Newman N, Hamed H, Fentiman IS, D'Arrigo C, Hanby AM, et al. Paget disease of the nipple. Cancer 2002;95(1):1–7.

[7] Sukumvanich P, Bentrem DJ, III HSC, Brogi E, Fey J V., Borgen PI, et al. The role of sentinel lymph node biopsy in Paget's disease of the breast. Ann Surg Oncol 2007;14(3):1020–3.

[8] Li Y-J, Huang X-E, Zhou X-D. Local breast cancer recurrence after mastectomy and breast-conserving surgery for Paget's disease: A meta-analysis. Breast Care 2014;9(6):431–4.

[9] Wong SM, Freedman RA, Stamell E, Sagara Y, Brock JE, Desantis SD, et al. Modern trends in the surgical management of Paget's disease. Ann Surg Oncol 2015;22(10):3308–16.

[10] Fisher B, Anderson S, Bryant J, Margolese RG, Deutsch M, Fisher ER, et al. Twenty-year follow-up of a randomized trial comparing total mastectomy, lumpectomy, and lumpectomy plus irradiation for the treatment of invasive breast cancer. N Engl J Med 2002;347(16):1233–41.

[11] Dixon AR, Galea MH, Ellis IO, Elston CW, Blamey RW. Paget's disease of the nipple. Br J Surg 1991;78(6):722–3.

[12] Marshall JK, Griffith KA, Haffty BG, Solin LJ, Vicini FA, McCormick B, et al. Conservative management of Paget disease of the breast with radiotherapy. Cancer 2003;97(9):2142–9.

SECTION THREE: BONE METASTASES AND HETEROTOPIC OSSIFICATION

In: Clinical Oncology
Editors: Ariel Tenenbaum et al.
ISBN: 978-1-53617-933-0

Chapter 6

PICTORIAL ESSAY OF RADIOLOGIC FINDINGS FOLLOWING PALLIATIVE TREATMENT FOR BONE METASTASES

Nicole Christakis[1], Bo Angela Wan[2], MD(C), Edward Chow[2] and Linda Probyn[1,*], MD
[1]Department of Diagnostic Imaging, Odette Cancer Centre, Sunnybrook Health Sciences Centre, University of Toronto, Toronto, Ontario, Canada
[2]Department of Radiation Oncology, Odette Cancer Centre, Sunnybrook Health Sciences Centre, University of Toronto, Toronto, Ontario, Canada

ABSTRACT

Bone is one of the most common sites of cancer metastases. Bone metastasis can lead to a variety of symptoms such as pain, bone fracture, and spinal cord compression that adversely affect patient quality of life. To prevent or ameliorate these symptoms, patients with bone metastasis are often treated palliatively with surgery, chemotherapy, radiation therapy or a combination of therapies. Imaging plays a vital role in

* Corresponding Author's E-mail: Linda.Probyn@sunnybrook.ca.

enabling the diagnosis, treatment, and monitoring of bone metastases. Following treatment there are many common radiologic findings.

INTRODUCTION

In this pictorial essay we will illustrate typical imaging appearances, responses of the tumors to treatment and also radiographic changes to the surrounding tissues secondary to treatment.

TUMOUR RESPONSE

Tumors can respond to chemotherapy or radiation either positively or may have no effect on the progression of disease. Figure 1 shows metastatic osteolytic lesions that positively respond to treatment with reactive bone, generally with new bone progressing from the periphery of the lesion (1).

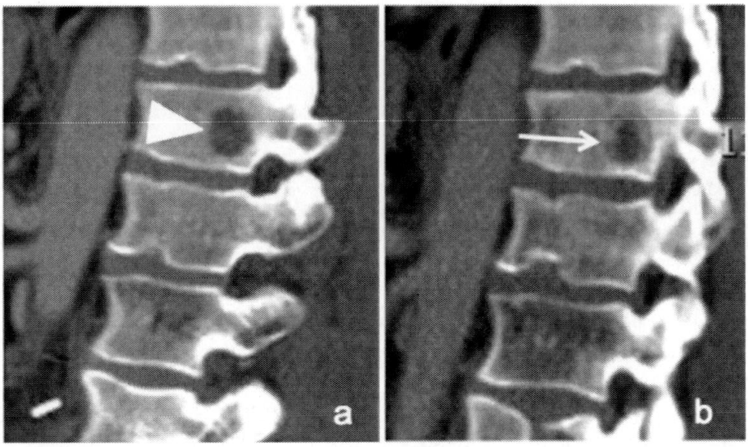

Figure 1. Sagittal CT images of the lumbar spine in a patient with metastatic renal cell carcinoma to the lumbar spine.In Figure 1a, there is an osteolytic lesion in the posterior aspect of the L1 vertebral body (white arrowhead). Figure 1b is 6 months treatment with Pazopanib, showing some reconstitution of the bone in the metastatic focus (white arrow).

On magnetic resonance (MR) imaging, normal bone marrow is predominantly fat and is high signal on T1W imaging. Metastatic infiltration generally appears as decreased signal on T1W images, reflecting replacement of the fat. Positive response to treatment can show reconstitution of normal marrow fat, as shown in Figure 2 (2).

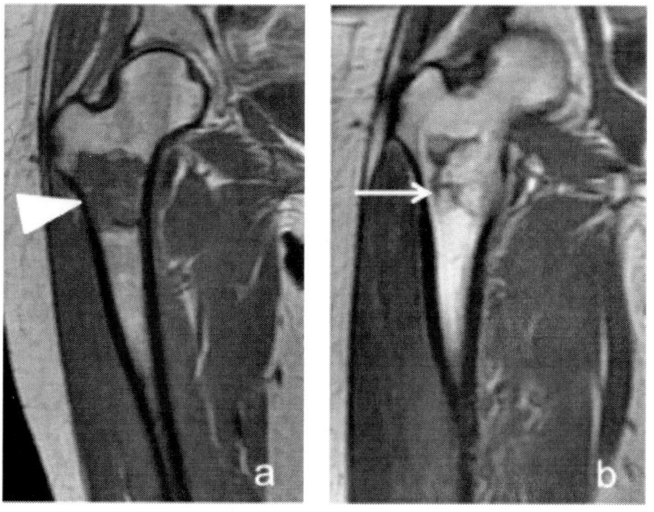

Figure 2. Coronal T1W images of the right femur in a patient with metastatic thyroid cancer. Figure 2a shows the initial MRI, demonstrating a large subtrochanteric lesion (white arrowhead). Following treatment (Figure 2b), there has been significant improvement with near complete reconstitution of normal marrow signal.

Effective treatment reduces metabolic tumor activity on positron-emission tomography (PET), whereas persistent abnormal uptake is usually associated with treatment failure, as shown in Figure 3 (3). Often, metastatic disease will progress despite treatment (Figures 4, 5).

Tumor cells are not the only cells to be destroyed by radiation therapy. Normal cells are also affected. This can be seen on imaging. On MR images, the exact extent of the radiation field can be seen. Within the radiation field, the bone marrow is fattier due to depletion of the hematopoietic cells and therefore demonstrates increase signal on the T1 images. At the edge of the radiation field, abrupt demarcation occurs at the margin with more normal appearing signal within the marrow outside of the radiated field as shown in Figure 6 (4).

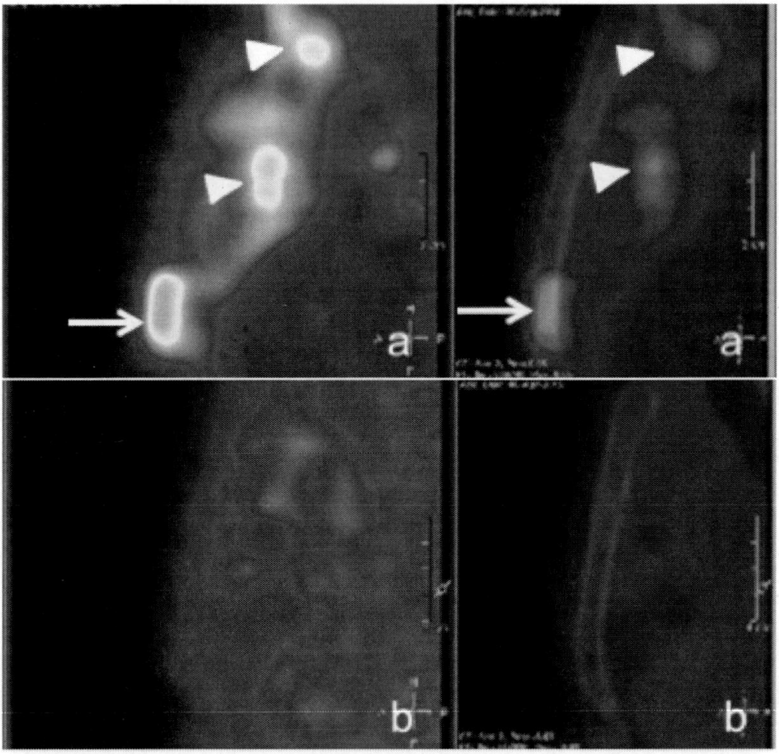

Figure 3. PET imaging of patient with Hodgkin's lymphoma with metastatic bone involvement in the distal sternum. Figure 3a shows Extensive mediastinal lymph node activity (arrowheads) and sternal activity (white arrow). Following radiation and chemotherapy (Figure 3b), no residual activity is present in the mediastinum or sternum.

Positron emission tomography is an imaging technique that is used to view the metabolic processes in the body. Fludeoxyglucose (FDG) is injected into a patient, where the body uses it like glucose. FDG-is a substance that is not chemically stable and releases energy which is detected by a special camera. Since the body's cells use FDG like glucose, activity on a PET scan shows tissues that are metabolically active. Various organs, tissues, and tumours are usually active, as shown in Figure 7 (3).

The manifestation of new or progressing bone lesions in patients responding to treatments may be incorrectly classified as progression of disease rather than a positive response. This is called the flare response. Increased activity on bone scans normally indicate progression of the disease, however the increased activity in flare response are the osteoclasts and osteoblasts functioning to repair bone following a positive response to treatment. A similar flare response can also be seen on radiographs or computed tomography (CT). This response is usually found during a short term follow up of lesions, where it would be unlikely for the disease to have progressed as shown on figures 8-10 (5).

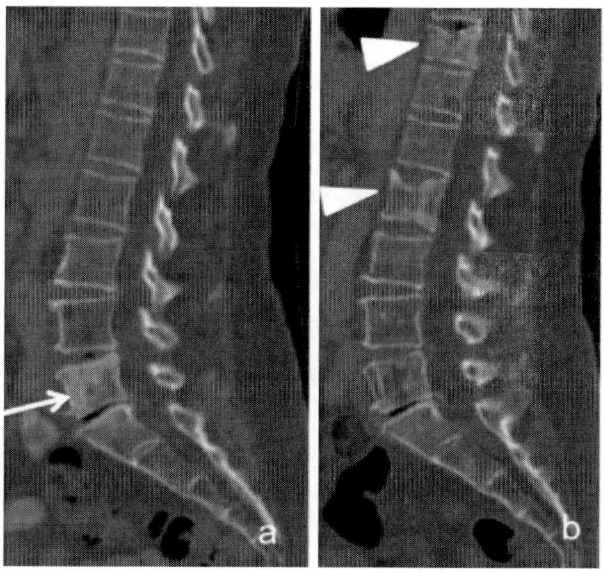

Figure 4. Sagittal reformatted CT images of the lumbar spine in a patient with metastatic breast carcinoma treated with Exemestane showing progressive metastatic disease despite treatment. Figure 4a demonstrates a mixed lytic and sclerotic metastatic focus in the L5 vertebral body (white arrow). Figure 4b shows that 8 months later on treatment, the patient has developed new lesions at T11 and L2 (white arrowheads) with pathologic fractures and depression of the superior endplates.

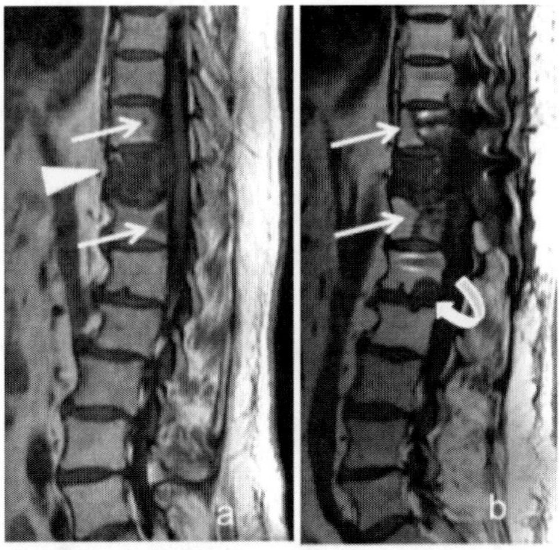

Figure 5. Sagittal T1W images of the lumbar spine 4 months apart following radiation treatment and surgery. Figure 5a of the initial image demonstrates dominant metastatic lesion in T11 vertebral body (arrowhead) and smaller lesions in the T10 and T12 vertebral bodies (white arrows). Figure 5b shows that following radiation and surgery, there was progression of the lesions in the T10 and T12 vertebral bodies and new lesion in the L1 vertebral body (curved arrow).

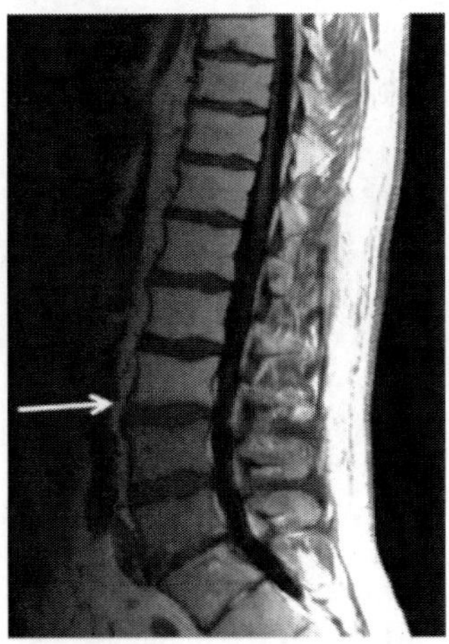

Figure 6. T1W sagittal image of the lumbar spine in a patient who has had previous radiation treatment. Arrow delineates the edge of the radiation field. The radiated vertebral levels cranial to the arrow demonstrate fatty replacement and increased T1W signal. Caudal to the radiation field the signal in the vertebral bodies is of normal hematopoietic marrow and therefore demonstrates relative decreased T1W signal.

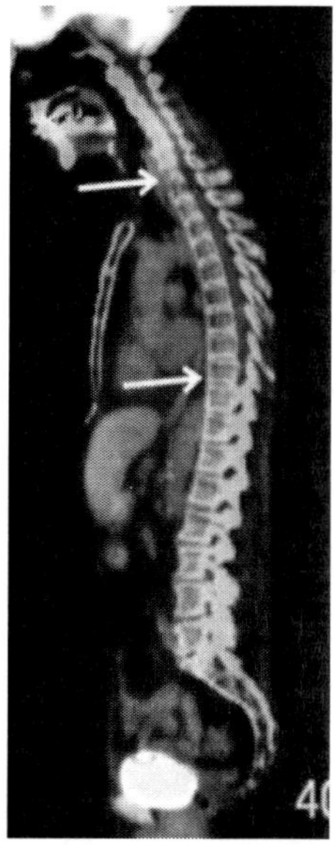

Figure 7. Sagittal PET image of the spine demonstrating decreased activity on PET in the radiation field (white arrows indicate margins of radiation field).

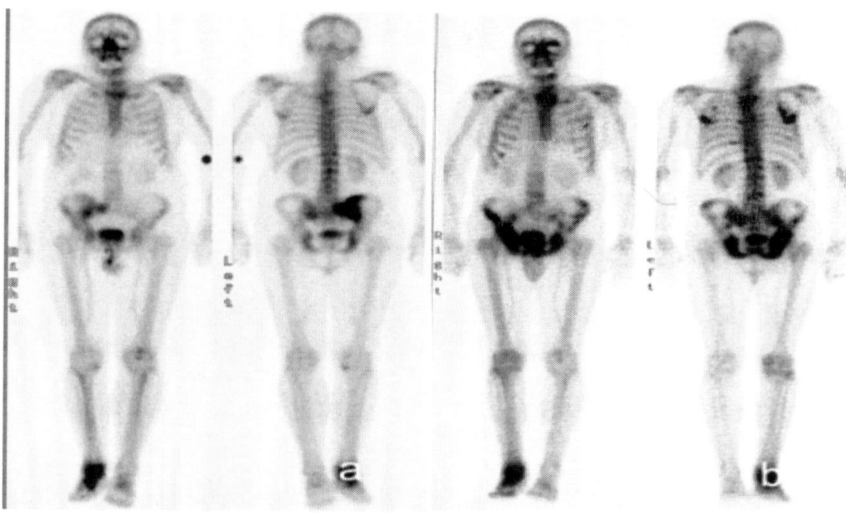

Figure 8. Flare response to chemotherapy in a patient with metastatic breast carcinoma to bone. Baseline bone scan is presented in Figure 8a, demonstrating increased activity predominantly in the pelvis. Figure 8b shows that 3 months after chemotherapy, there is increased activity within the pelvis and multiple new areas in the ribs and spine.

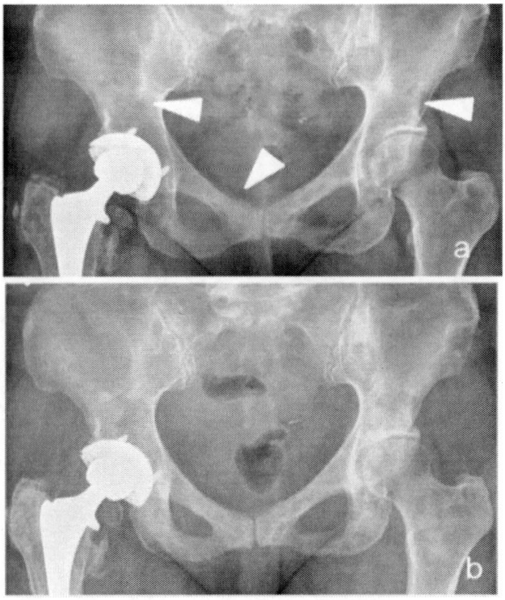

Figure 9. Flare AP pelvis in a patient with metastatic breast carcinoma.
Figure 9a shows diffuse mixed lytic and sclerotic metastatic foci throughout the pelvis and proximal left femur (arrowheads indicating some of the lesions). Figure 9b shows that 3 months after chemotherapy, there is increased size and number of sclerotic lesions in keeping with a flare response.

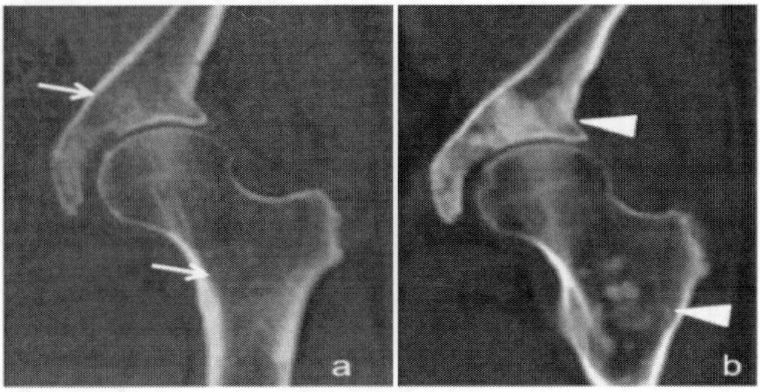

Figure 10. Flare response to treatment show in coronal reformatted CT images of a hip in a patient with diffuse metastatic breast carcinoma. Figure 10a of pre-treatment CT shows very subtle marrow soft tissue density in the acetabulum and proximal femur (arrows). Figure 10b of 2 months post chemotherapy shows increased sclerosis in the acetabulum and femur which could be misinterpreted as progression of disease but represents a positive response to treatment with reactive sclerosis (arrowheads).

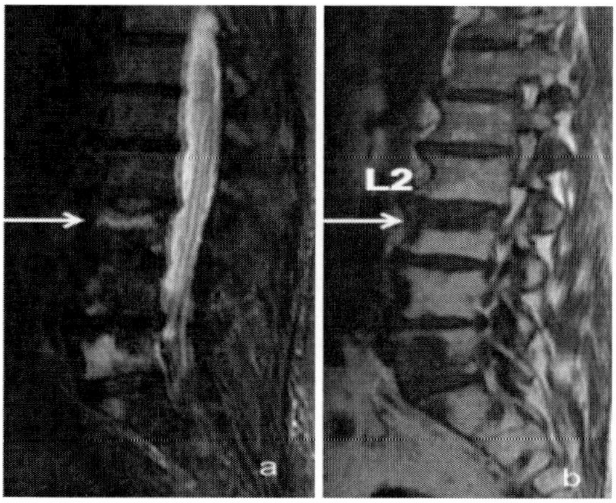

Figure 11. Patient with metastatic melanoma. Figure 11a shows a sagittal STIR MR image, and Figure 11b shows a sagittal T1W MR image. Radiation therapy to was used to treat the lumbar spine. Note the fatty change in the marrow caudal to L2 on the T1W image. There is an insufficiency fracture in the radiated bone of the superior endplate at L3 (white arrow) with depression of the endplate and linear abnormal signal paralleling the endplate.

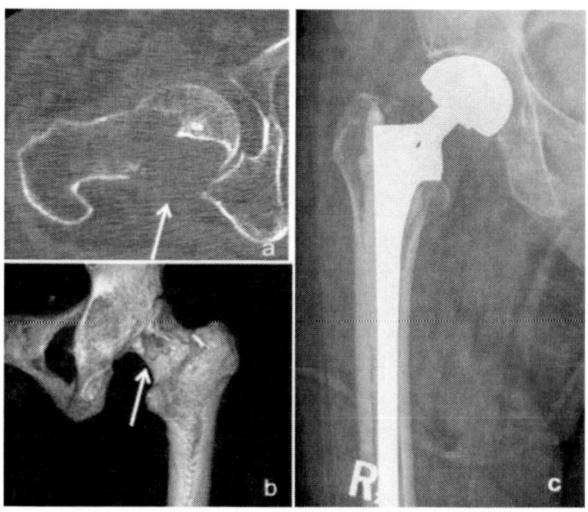

Figure 12. Osteolytic metastatic lesion in the right femoral neck and prophylactic cemented hemiarthroplasty. Figure 12a is an axial CT image. Figure 12b is a 3D CT image. Patient has an osteolytic metastatic lesion in the right femoral neck with cortical destruction posteriorly (white arrows) at high risk for pathologic fracture. Figure 10c is a radiograph that shows the postoperative appearance of a prophylactic cemented hemiarthroplasty.

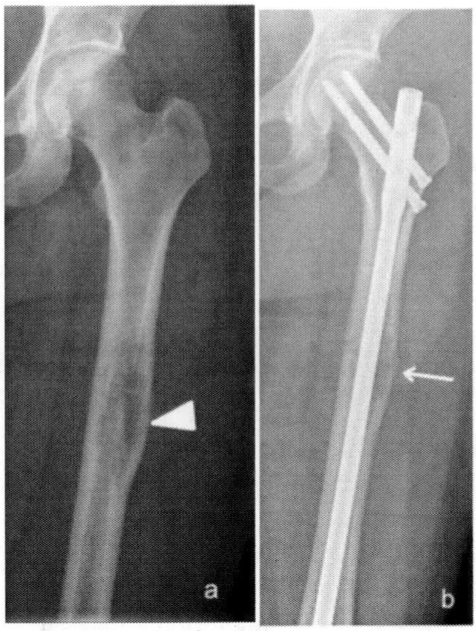

Figure 13. Patient with metastatic breast carcinoma. Figure 13a shows a large osteolytic lesion in the proximal femoral shaft (white arrowhead) with significant cortical permeation and destruction at very high risk of fracture. Figure 13b shows intramedullary rod placement for fracture prophylaxis. A fracture (white arrow) developed during placement of the rod confirming the fragility of the femur secondary to the metastatic focus.

An insufficiency fracture occurs when weakened bone that is demineralized and has decreased elastic resistance is subjected to normal or physiological stress. Radiation affects mature bone by weakening its structural integrity and makes it more susceptible to stress fractures, as shown in Figure 11 (6).

Pathologic fractures occur as a result of weakening of the mechanical properties of bone. Bony destruction by metastatic disease may result in pathologic fracture. The risk of sustaining a pathological fracture through a metastatic deposit in a long bone is predicted by the site of lesion, nature of lesion and degree of cortical destruction, size of lesion and pain (7). When the risk is high, prophylactic surgical stabilization is performed (Figures 12, 13).

Surgery is performed on the spine when the tumour in the spine is compressing or at risk for compressing the spinal cord. The posterior elements are often resected to alleviate pressure on the spinal cord, as shown in Figure 14 (8).

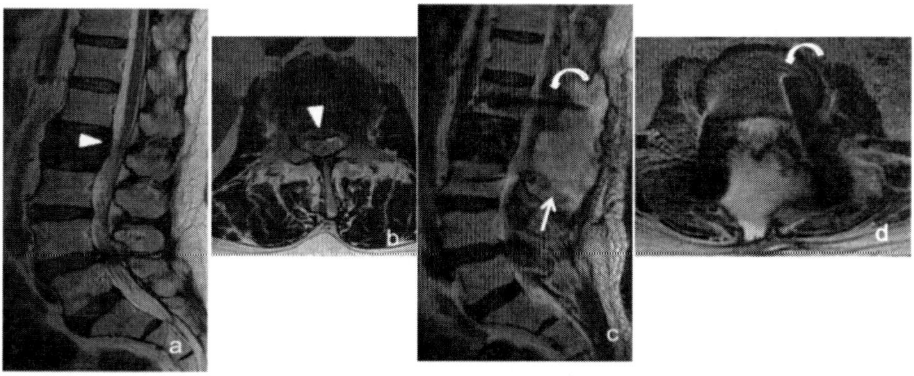

Figure 14. Patient with metastatic lung cancer to L2. Figure 14a is a sagittal image, and Figure 14b is an axial T2W image, demonstrating marrow replacement at L2 with extraosseous soft tissue posterior to the vertebral body and mild canal compromise (arrowheads). Figure 14c is a sagittal T2W image and Figure 14d is an axial T2W image following posterior decompression and instrumentation showing a large post-operative seroma/hematoma in the laminectomy (arrow) and posterior instrumentation (curved arrow).

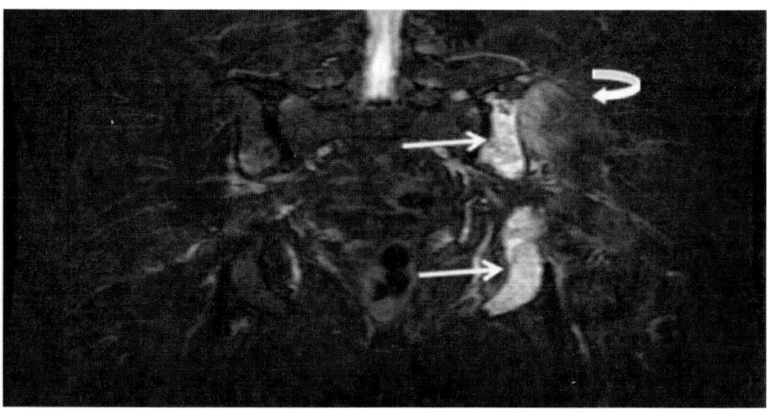

Figure 15. Coronal STIR MRI image of patients with bone metastasis who underwent radiation therapy. Metastasis in the left ilium and ischium (white arrows). Feathery increased T2W signal in the left gluteal muscles (curved arrow) secondary to radiation changes.

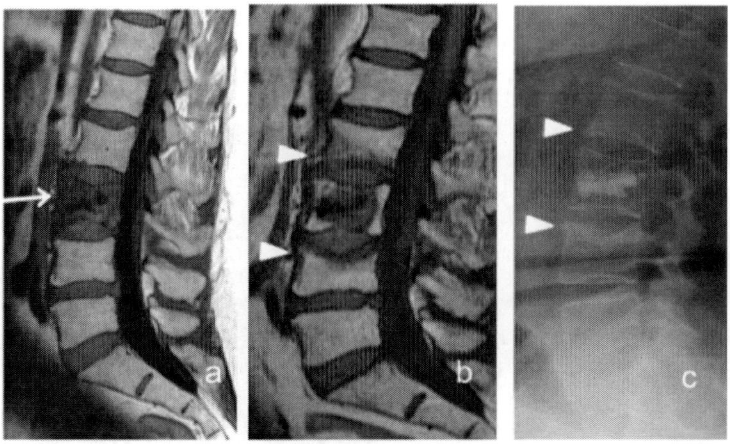

Figure 16. Patient with metastatic renal cell carcinoma to the L3 vertebral body with vertebroplasty. Figure 16a shows the vertebroplasty at L3. The sagittal T1W image demonstrates the very low signal cement in the L3 vertebral body metastatic focus (straight arrow). Figure 16b is a saggital T1W image at 4 months post vertebroplasty, depicting new endplate fractures in the inferior aspect of L2 and superior aspect of L4 (arrowheads). Figure 16c is a lateral radiograph demonstrating the same endplate fractures (arrowheads).

Radiation can cause vasculitis and muscle cell injury which can result in increased extracellular fluid in muscle. This manifests as increased T2W signal in the muscles confined to the radiation field. The abrupt lateral margin of the abnormal increased signal corresponds to the radiation field. This abnormal muscle signal will resolve over time, as shown in Figure 15 (9).

When a patient has an osteolytic bone lesion that is at risk for fracture or has fractured they can have a cementoplasty (packing bone with cement), which includes procedures such as vertebroplasty, kyphoplasty, osteoplasty, and sacroplasty. These procedures strive to treat or prevent pathological fractures and pain in patients with vertebral and extra spinal osteolytic lesions. The cement is dense on radiographs or CT and shows low signal on all MRI sequences. Delayed complications are that the patient may develop fractures at the next vertebral level because of altered biomechanics. The cement is very hard and increases the stiffness of the vertebral body. This may result in increased force loading on the adjacent vertebral bodies and result in fracture, as show in Figure 16 (10).

The lung is particularly sensitive to radiation. Initially, the radiation damages the lung epithelium and causes inflammation. This then stimulates fibroblasts to produce collagen which results in chronic permanent fibrotic changes, as shown in Figure 17 (11).

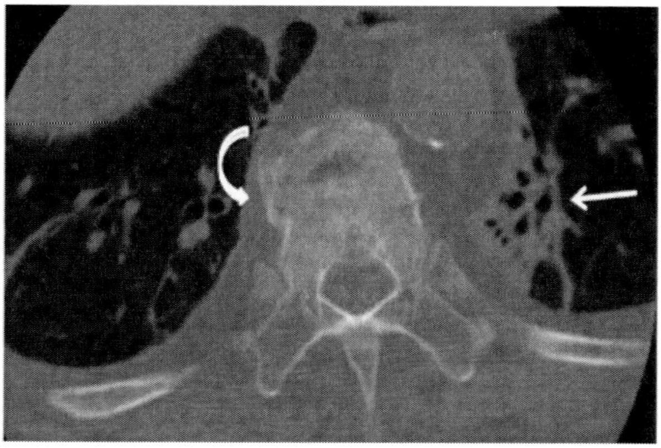

Figure 17. Axial CT image of the thoracic spine in a patient with metastatic prostate carcinoma treated with radiation 6 months ago.
Fibrosis and bronchiectasis in the adjacent lung with a discrete lateral border corresponding to the radiation field in the adjacent lung (white arrow). Diffuse sclerotic metastatic lesion in the adjacent vertebral body (curved arrow).

CONCLUSION

Imaging plays an integral part in diagnosis of bone metastases and follow-up after treatment. Knowledge of the tumor response, appearance of treatment material, changes in the surrounding tissues and complications on various imaging modalities is important to properly further manage these cancer patients.

REFERENCES

[1] Rybak LD, Rosenthal DI. Radiological imaging for the diagnosis of bone metastases. Q J Nucl Med 2001;45(1):53-64.

[2] Hamaoka T, Madewell JE, Podoloff DA, Hortobagyi GN, Ueno NT. Bone imaging in metastatic breast cancer. J Clin Oncol 2004;22(14):2942-53.

[3] Kazama T, Faria SC, Varavithya V, Phongkitkarun S, Ito H, Macapinlac HA. FDG PET in the evaluation of treatment for lymphoma: Clinical usefulness and pitfalls. Radiographics 2005;25(1):191-207.

[4] Ramsey RG, Zacharias CE. MR imaging of the spine after radiation therapy: easily recognizable effects. AJR Am J Roentgenol 1985;144(6):1131-5.

[5] Messiou C, Cook G, Reid AH, Attard G, Dearnaley D, de Bono JS, et al. The CT flare response of metastatic bone disease in prostate cancer. Acta Radiol 2011;52(5):557-61.

[6] Oh D, Huh SJ. Insufficiency fracture after radiation therapy. Radiat Oncol J 2014;32(4):213-20

[7] Kornah B, Safwat H, Ghany TA, AAl MA, Saleem N. Prophylactic fixation of impending fractures. MOJ Orthop Rheumatol 2016;6(1):00206

[8] Tanaka M, Nakahara S, Ito Y, Kunisada T, Misawa H, Koshimune K, et al. Surgical treatment of metastatic vertebral tumors. Acta Med Okayama 2009;63(3):145-50.

[9] McMahon CJ, Wu JS, Eisenberg RL. Muscle edema. AJR Am J Roentgenol 2010;194(4):284-92.

[10] Gu YF, Li YD, Wu CG, Sun ZK, He CJ. Safety and efficacy of percutaneous vertebroplasty and interventional tumor removal for metastatic spinal tumors and malignant vertebral compression fractures. AJR Am J Roentgenol 2014;202(3):298-305.

[11] Choi YW, Munden RF, Erasmus JJ, Park KJ, Chung WK, Jeon SC, et al. Effects of radiation therapy on the lung: radiologic appearances and differential diagnosis. Radiographics 2004;24(4):985-97.

In: Clinical Oncology
Editors: Ariel Tenenbaum et al.
ISBN: 978-1-53617-933-0

Chapter 7

TIBIAL METASTASIS AS A PRESENTING SYMPTOM OF ENDOMETRIAL ADENOCARCINOMA: A CASE REPORT

Caitlin Yee, Bo Angela Wan, MD(C), Linda Probyn, MD, Vithusha Ganesh, MD(C), Leah Drost, Akanksha Kulshreshtha, MD(C), Rashi Asthana, MSc, Edward Chow, and Elizabeth Barnes*, MD

Odette Cancer Centre, Sunnybrook Health Sciences Centre,
University of Toronto, Toronto, Ontario, Canada

ABSTRACT

Bone metastases below the knee are rare, but when they occur they often present challenges to the patient's mobility and ability to perform

* Corresponding Author: Elizabeth Barnes, MD, FRCPC, Department of Radiation Oncology, Odette Cancer Centre, Sunnybrook Health Sciences Centre, 2075 Bayview Avenue, Toronto ON, Canada. E-mail: toni.barnes@sunnybrook.ca.

activities of daily living. We report the case of a 54-year-old woman who presented with tibial and lung metastases at the time of her diagnosis of an endometrial adenocarcinoma. The patient was treated with radiation therapy, surgery to stabilize the tibia, and systemic chemotherapy. Although treatment was initially effective in palliating symptoms, at the time of the most recent follow-up, 19 months after her initial diagnosis, the patient's pain had returned to her left tibia. Because of the limited number of similar cases reported in the literature, the prognosis for patients with endometrial carcinoma presenting with below-the-knee bone metastases is not well understood.

INTRODUCTION

Bone metastases in the appendicular skeleton are rare (less than 15% of all cases), and are generally associated with primary cancer sites in the lung, liver, prostate, thyroid, or breast (1, 2). They most commonly appear on the femur or humerus (1, 2). Although metastatic disease to bone is rare in cases of endometrial cancer (3–5), the proportion of metastases occurring below the knee appears to be higher in this population. In a literature review conducted by Boukhar et al. 28% of bone metastases in patients with endometrial carcinoma were found on the tibia and bones of the foot (4). Below-the-knee metastases can severely diminish the patient's quality of life (QoL), since they often affect weight-bearing bones such as the tibia, leading to decreased mobility and function (1).

This report presents the case of a 54-year-old woman with an anterior tibial lesion and lung nodules upon diagnosis of endometrial adenocarcinoma.

CASE STORY

In December of 2015, a 54-year-old woman presented to the emergency room with pain in the left anterior tibia. The patient was healthy apart from a history of a benign thyroid nodule, with no family history of malignancy and no previous diagnosis of cancer. She had been experiencing postmenopausal bleeding since November 2015. An ultrasound Doppler of the left lower extremity was conducted, but no vascular abnormalities were found. The leg pain went away without treatment. The leg pain returned in January 2016, at which point an x-ray was taken and a lytic lesion measuring 6 x 0.9 cm was discovered on the anterior aspect of the left tibia (see Figure 1). Magnetic resonance imaging (MRI) of the left lower limb showed an aggressive-appearing lesion involving the mid-tibia measuring 5.7 x 2.9 x 2 cm (see Figure 2). A bone scan showed uptake in the left mid-third tibia shaft. An open biopsy showed metastatic adenocarcinoma, with immunohistochemical staining consistent with a gynecological origin. Metastatic workup was conducted including a pelvic ultrasound revealing an enlarged uterus (10 x 7.3 x 6.3 cm) and ovaries (R: 4.2 x 3.4 x 3 cm, L: 5.7, 4.4, 3.4 cm). A computerized tomography (CT) scan showed two nodular foci in the right upper lobe of the lung measuring 4 mm that were suspected to be malignant.

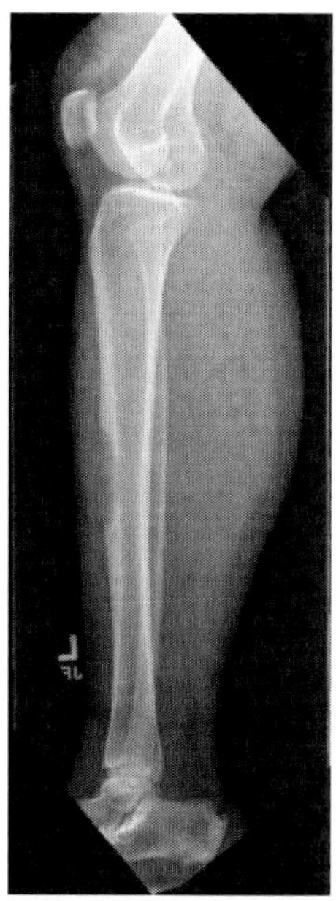

Figure 1. Lateral X-ray of left tibia and fibula demonstrating a destructive osteolytic lesion in the anterior aspect of the mid tibial shaft. Given the extent of involvement there is a high risk of pathologic fracture.

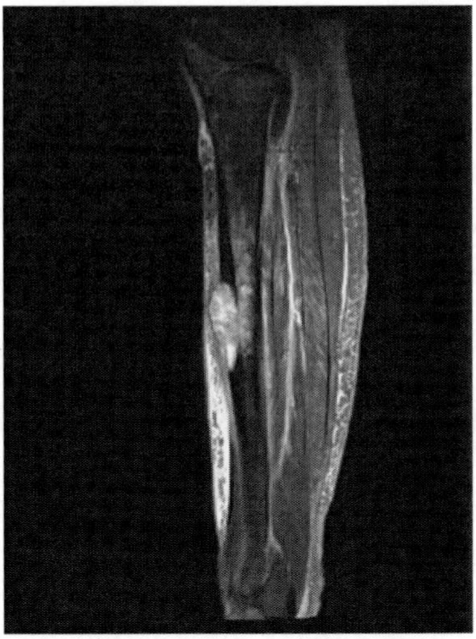

Figure 2. MRI of left leg taken in December 2016. Sagittal T2 fat suppressed MR image of the tibia demonstrating a destructive soft tissue mass in the anterior mid tibial shaft with extra-osseous soft tissue extension that is heterogeneous and predominately high signal. There is high signal abnormality in the marrow and soft tissue edema.

The patient received palliative radiotherapy 30 Gy in 10 fractions to the left tibia in April 2016. Prior to treatment the patient was taking one or two Percocet per day. The patient felt that radiotherapy was effective in relieving her leg pain, although she experienced some swelling of the thigh and abdominal cramps for which she took Tylenol-2. She continued to experience vaginal bleeding, and was initially scheduled for a hysterectomy in late July. However, the patient was admitted to hospital in June with severe pain (10/10) in her left buttock radiating down the left leg, and urinary retention requiring catheter placement. CT imaging found a large (4 x 4.3 cm) destructive bony lesion invading the left sacrum and S2-4 neural foramina. The hysterectomy was cancelled at this time, as it was not expected to significantly improve her quality of life. The patient instead received 30 Gy in 10 fractions of radiotherapy to the pelvis to encompass the sacral disease and the uterus. This reduced her pain, reversed her neurologic compromise, improved her mobility and stopped her vaginal bleeding. She was also started on medroxyprogesterone.

In December 2016, the patient returned with mild pain and erythema on the anterior aspect of her left tibia. MRI showed a destructive tibial lesion (11.1 cm in length) with a large soft tissue component and a smaller skip lesion in the proximal tibial shaft (see Figure 3-5). Referral was made to an orthopaedic surgeon, as the tibia was determined to be at high risk of fracture. The patient underwent an elective prophylactic surgery in January 2017 with intramedullary nailing of the left tibia. This was followed by postoperative radiotherapy of 25 Gy in 10 fractions. Her pain improved post treatment. The medroxyprogesterone was stopped, and from March-July 2017, the patient received 6 cycles of doxorubicin and carboplatin. Repeat imaging shows no progression of systemic disease; however she has slowly progressive pain in her left tibia. The patient continues to attend regular follow-up appointments with her physicians.

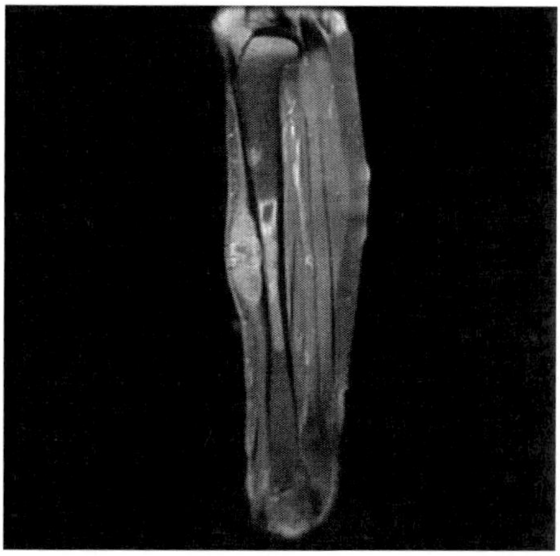

Figure 3. MRI of left leg taken July 2017. Sagittal T1 fat suppressed post gadolinium (Figure 3), Sagittal T1 (Figure 4) and axial T2 fat suppressed (Figure 5) MR images demonstrates progression of the large destructive soft tissue mass in the anterior mid tibial shaft with increased extra-osseous soft tissue. There is low T1 signal, intermediate to increased T2 signal and enhancement post-gadolinium. There is a skip lesion in the proximal tibial shaft not present previously.

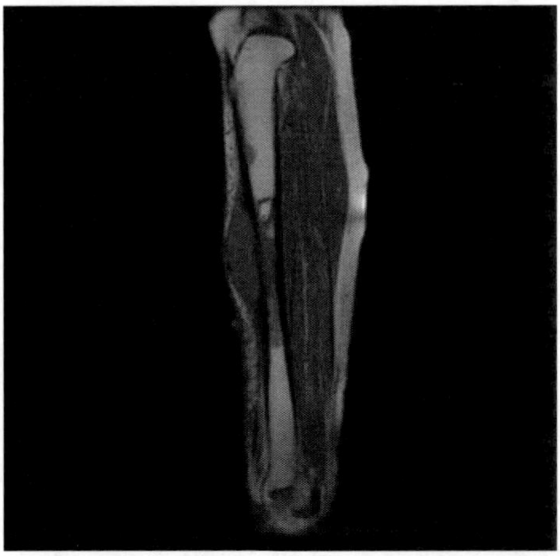

Figure 4. MRI of left leg taken July 2017, alternate view.

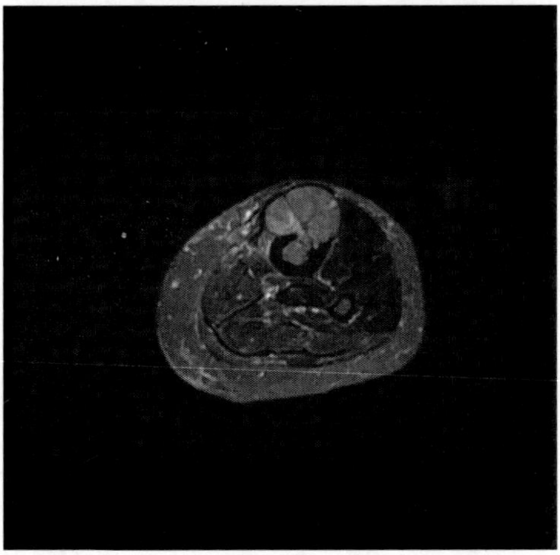

Figure 5. MRI of left leg taken July 2017, cross-sectional view.

DISCUSSION

In approximately 90% of women with endometrial cancer, the first sign of disease is abnormal vaginal bleeding (4). 72% of endometrial cancers are discovered while they are still confined to the uterus and prognosis is very good for this population (4). This patient had the unusual presentation of tibial and lung metastases at initial diagnosis. Lung is a common metastatic site, but bone metastases rare in endometrial cancer (3).

A major concern with below-the-knee metastases is the impact on the patient's mobility and QoL (1). This patient experienced severe pain which seriously interfered with her activities of daily living. The lesion on her tibia also presented a significant fracture risk, which required surgery to stabilize. The patient was given an additional 25 Gy in 10 fractions of radiation therapy following surgery. Postoperative radiation has been shown in cases such as these to decrease the probability of the patient requiring secondary surgery (6, 7).

Radiation therapy is the common treatment method for bone metastases, and has been shown to effectively palliate symptoms (5, 8). Combinations of radiotherapy, chemotherapy, surgery, and hormone therapy are often used to treat bone metastases, depending on the specific tumor type and presentation (2, 4, 8, 9). The patient described in this report completed a total of three courses of radiotherapy in addition to systemic chemotherapy, all of which were well-tolerated by the patient and effective in treating her symptoms.

Outcomes for patients with metastatic bone disease are generally poor (2). The patient discussed in the present case was not diagnosed until her disease had progressed to her lungs as well as her bones, and her treatment intent was therefore palliative rather than curative. At her most recent follow up, 19 months after her initial diagnosis, the patient was stable but continued to experience pain in her left tibia. A literature review by Kaya et al. identified 19 reported cases of endometrial carcinoma that metastasized to bone, and concluded that patients presenting with isolated skeletal metastases in early stages of the disease could possibly represent a population with above average prognoses and survival rates (3). Contrarily, a review by Kehoe et al. looked at 21 cases of patients diagnosed with bone metastases from endometrial cancer, and found that their prognosis was poor (8). This patient has survived 19 months from her initial diagnosis. Although her systemic disease is stable, she remains symptomatic from her tibial disease. Repeat imaging is pending and clinical trials may be a future treatment option.

Conclusion

This patient presented with a case of endometrial adenocarcinoma which had metastasized to her tibia and lung at the time of diagnosis, and developed sacral metastases within months. The patient was treated with radiation therapy, hormonal therapy and chemotherapy, standard treatments for bone metastases (8). The patient also had prophylactic surgery to stabilize her tibia, which was at risk of fracture. Because cases such as this are so uncommon, it is difficult to draw conclusions about optimal treatment and prognosis - more research is required to better understand the implications of this diagnosis. In this case, although treatment was initially effective in palliating the patient's symptoms she continued to experience pain at the site of her tibial metastasis 7 months after surgery and 19 months after diagnosis. Below-the-knee metastases can be difficult to treat, as pain in the weight-bearing bones of the lower limb compromises the patient's mobility.

Acknowledgments

We thank the generous support of Bratty Family Fund, Michael and Karyn Goldstein Cancer Research Fund, Joey and Mary Furfari Cancer Research Fund, Pulenzas Cancer Research Fund, Joseph and Silvana Melara Cancer Research Fund, and Ofelia Cancer Research Fund.

References

[1] Choi M, Probyn L, Rowbottom L, McDonald R, Bobrowski A, Chan S, et al. Clinical presentations of below knee bone metastases: A case series. Ann Palliat Med 2017;6.

[2] Söylemez MS, Kemah B, Söylemez UPO, Kılıç B, Ozkan K. Endometrial adenocarcinoma recurrence presenting with tibial metastasis: Report of a case. Int J Surg Case Rep 2017;36:15–7.

[3] Kaya A, Olmezoglu A, Eren CS, Bayol U, Altay T, Karapinar L, et al. Solitary bone metastasis in the tibia as a presenting sign of endometrial adenocarcinoma: a case report and the review of the literature. Clin Exp Metastasis 2007;24(2):87–92.

[4] Boukhar SA, Kaneshiro R, Schiller A, Terada K, Tauchi-Nishi P. Tibial bone metastasis as an initial presentation of endometrial carcinoma diagnosed by fine-needle aspiration cytology: A case report and review of the literature. Cytojournal 2015;12(11):4–9.

[5] Ishibashi M, Fujiwaki R, Nakayama I, Miura H, Sawada K. Endometrial carcinosarcoma presenting as a tibial metastasis. Int J Clin Oncol 2007;12(4):305–8.

[6] Drost L, Ganesh V, Wan BA, Raman S, Chan S, Christakis M, et al. Efficacy of postoperative radiation treatment for bone metastases in the extremities. Radiother Oncol 2017;124(1):45–8.

[7] Townsend PW, Smalley SR, Cozad SC, Rosenthal HG, Hassanein RES. Role of postoperative radiation therapy after stabilization of fractures caused by metastatic disease. Int J Radiat Oncol Biol Phys 1993;27(April):59–66.

[8] Kehoe SM, Zivanovic O, Ferguson SE, Barakat RR, Soslow RA. Clinicopathologic features of bone metastases and outcomes in patients with primary endometrial cancer. Gynecol Oncol 2010;117(2):229–33.

[9] Doger E, Cakiroglu Y, Ozdamar O, Ceylan Y, Kole E, Yucesoy I, et al. Bone metastasis in endometrial cancer: evaluation of treatment approaches by factors affecting prognosis. Eur J Gynaecol Oncol 2016;37(3):407–16.

In: Clinical Oncology
Editors: Ariel Tenenbaum et al.
ISBN: 978-1-53617-933-0

Chapter 8

RAPID FORMATION OF SIGNIFICANT HETEROTOPIC OSSIFICATION IN A CRITICALLY ILL PATIENT WITH NECROTIZING PANCREATITIS

Mary Jiayi Tao, MD, Linda Probyn, MD, Michael Poon, MD, Hans Kreder, MD, Bo Angela Wan and Edward Chow *

Odette Cancer Centre, Sunnybrook Health Sciences Centre, University of Toronto, Toronto, Ontario, Canada

ABSTRACT

Heterotopic ossification (HTO) is the dystrophic formation of mature lamellar bone outside the confines of normal osseous tissues. It is frequently a complication of traumatic insult, both iatrogenic and non-iatrogenic, in addition to neurological compromise. Predisposing risk factors for HTO formation include male gender, diffuse idiopathic skeletal hyperostosis, ankylosing spondylitis, immobilization, mechanical

* Corresponding Author's E-mail: Edward.Chow@sunnybrook.ca.

ventilation, and inflammation. Typically, such pathological osseous development occurs over several months before it becomes radiologically detectable. In this article, we present a case of accelerated formation of significant heterotopic ossifications just one month following a major motor vehicle accident in the setting of necrotizing pancreatitis followed by a brief review of the multifactorial nature of such rapid progression of disease.

INTRODUCTION

Heterotopic ossification (HTO) is the pathological formation of mature lamellar bone in non-osseous tissues. While this process most commonly occurs in the skin, subcutaneous tissues, skeletal muscles, connective tissues, and nerves, it has been described within blood vessel walls and the mesenteries in rare cases (1). The development of ectopic bone can lead to significant joint stiffness, functional limitations, painful impingements and an overall reduction in quality of life. A major predisposing factor for HTO is inciting trauma while inflammation is known to play an important role as it often stimulates osteoprogenitor cell proliferation (2).

The histological development of post-traumatic heterotopic ossification begins with spindle cell proliferation during the first week followed by primitive osteoid formation in the second week (3). Although radiographs may detect scattered circumferential ossification with lucent centers as early as 4-6 weeks, it is typically only after six months where the formation of extra-osseous tissues can truly be appreciated radiographically (1, 3).

We describe a case with the accelerated development of significant heterotopic ossifications just one month following a major motor vehicle accident.

CASE STORY

A previously healthy 29-year-old male was transferred to our institution from a peripheral hospital after being involved in a high-speed motor vehicle accident. At the time of initial assessment, the only detectable injury was a right posterior acetabular fracture-dislocation which was concentrically reduced at the community hospital. He was subsequently brought to our institution for definitive fracture fixation at three days following his initial injury. Shortly after the induction of general anesthesia, he become febrile and tachycardic with an increased end-tidal carbon dioxide. As a result, the operation was aborted on the presumptive diagnosis of malignant hyperthermia. He was adequately resuscitated and transferred to the intensive care unit (ICU) in stable condition.

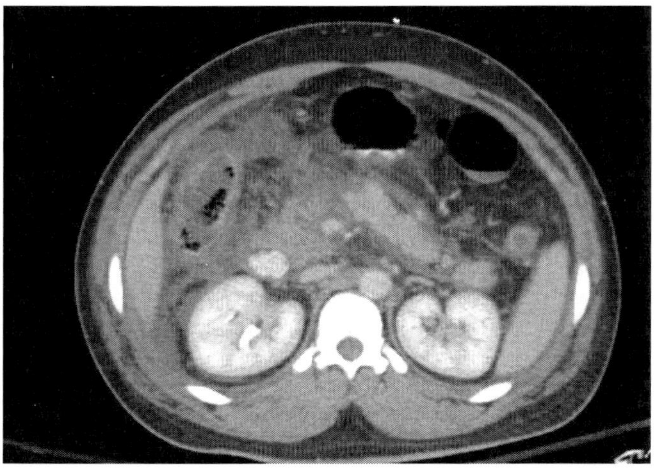

Figure 1. Axial intravenously enhanced image through the abdomen demonstrating a pancreatic transection with surround peripancreatic fluid and inflammatory stranding.

Over the course of his ICU stay, his abdomen became increasingly distended and he rapidly deteriorated. CT scan of the abdomen/pelvis demonstrated a complete pancreatic transection at the level of the neck and body with extensive peripancreatic stranding and edema (Figure 1). He was taken to the operating room the same day for urgent exploratory laparotomy with appropriate precautionary measures for malignant hyperthermia. Intraoperatively, there was significant pancreatic necrosis with surrounding inflammation. A distal pancreatectomy was not completed given the significant risk of bleeding. Instead three Jackson-Pratt drains were inserted to facilitate for post-operative washout to control the extent of inflammation and necrosis. Overall, he tolerated the procedure well without any perioperative complications.

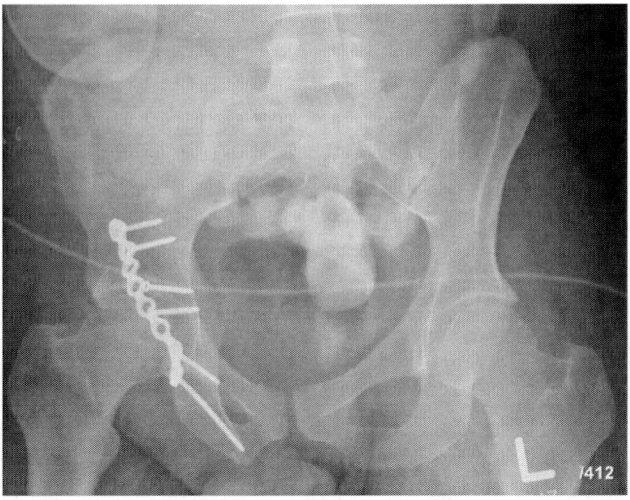

Figure 2. Immediate postoperative plain radiograph of the pelvis after open reduction and internal fixation of a right acetabular fracture with reconstruction plate fixation. Overall anatomical alignment is maintained.

The patient remained in the ICU with mechanical ventilatory support for several days before he was deemed stable enough to undergo another operation. Two days later, he was brought back into the operating room for definitive fixation of the acetabular fracture-dislocation using a posterior Kocher-Langenbeck approach. He tolerated the procedure well without any immediate complications. Post-operative radiographs are seen in Figure 2.

Over the course of the next two weeks, he improved clinically and was transferred to a community hospital in stable condition. He was instructed to not weight-bear on his right lower extremity until further assessment.

At the one-month follow-up, the patient had restricted hip range of motion with little pain. Compared to the radiographs taken on the day of the operation, there is newly developed heterotopic ossifications of significant caliber immediately superior to the right hip (Figure 3). Despite adequate physiotherapy, the patient continued to experience limited abduction and minimal rotation over the next year. Radiographs confirmed the presence of extensive right hip HTO (Figure 4). As a result, surgical resection was performed with postoperative prophylactic irradiation.

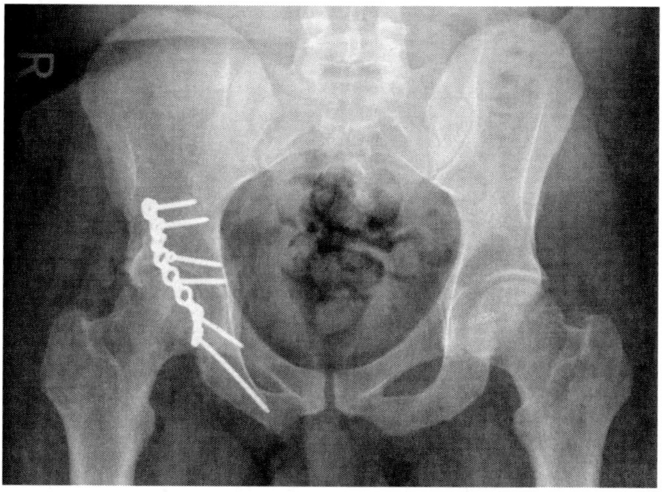

Figure 3. Plain radiograph of the pelvis one month after open reduction and internal fixation of a right acetabular fracture with developing heterotopic ossification at the superior aspect of the right hip.

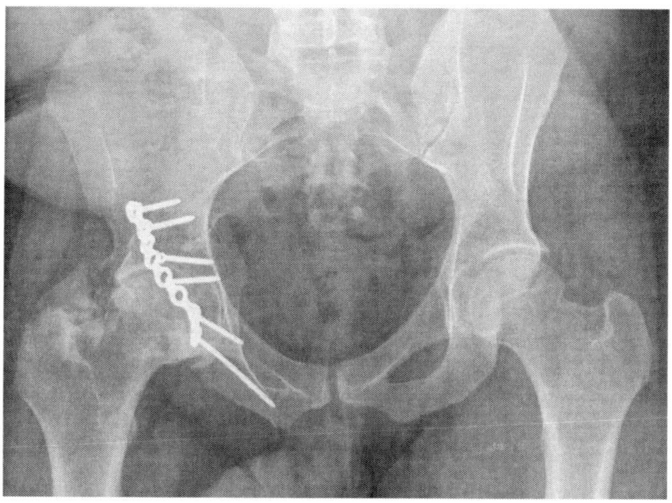

Figure 4. Plain radiograph of the pelvis demonstrating maturing heterotopic ossification at the superior aspect of the right hip one year following the operation.

Discussion

Heterotopic ossification affects a considerable proportion of critically ill patients as it has been associated with acute respiratory distress syndrome (ARDS), paralysis and immobilization, head and spinal cord injuries, prolonged mechanical ventilation, pancreatitis and burns (4). In a study conducted by Slutsky et al., it was shown that five percent of patients in the ICU with underlying ARDS had enlargement and immobility of large joints secondary to heterotopic ossification (5). Typically, the formation of such lesions occurs over a period of several months; however, this study describes a case in which clinically significant heterotopic ossifications formed over the course of one month in the setting of traumatic injury and necrotizing pancreatitis. While the exact mechanism for such rapid progression remains speculative, it is likely that a variety of triggers including inflammation, mechanical ventilation, surgical approach, immobilization and lack of prophylactic measures all played an important role in facilitating such an accelerated development.

Bone morphogenetic proteins (BMPs) are key mediators in the physiological formation of bone tissue. On the other hand, overexpression of BMPs is potentially pathological as it may induce the otherwise dormant osteoprogenitor mesenchymal stem cells to differentiate into bone through the endochondral pathway in para-articular soft tissues (6). Inflammation is known to be a predisposing factor in this progression as TNFα stimulates the expression of BMPs in addition to augmenting muscle-residing stroma cells (mrSCs) which acts to enhance bone formation (7). While there are numerous pro-inflammatory triggers, immobilization significantly potentiates this state in the setting of critically ill patients given the extensive disuse atrophy and muscle loss associated with prolonged intensive care unit stays (8). Additionally, although necrotizing pancreatitis has not been independently linked with heterotopic ossification, it is an extremely inflammatory process which releases humoral factors that induce surrounding hypoxia and edema. Furthermore, previous studies have also demonstrated that sedation and mechanical ventilation may induce respiratory alkalosis which will consequently alternate the local tissue pH and oxygenation (9, 10). This will in turn change the precipitation kinetics of calcium and phosphate salts to result in a permissive environment for pathological bone development (11).

Several surgical factors may have precipitated the rapid progression of heterotopic ossification in our patient. Firstly, the delay in surgical intervention may have impacted the extent of disease it has been shown that the time interval between the initial traumatic injury and definitive surgery is a significant predicator in the formation of symptomatic heterotopic ossification (12). Additionally, the choice in surgical approach is an important consideration. In a small retrospective review concluded by Russell et al., it was found that patients who underwent the direct anterior approach for total hip arthroplasties (THA) were significantly less likely to develop clinically significant ossifications compared to those who underwent the posterior approach (13). Such observation may be explained by the reduced soft-tissue trauma associated with the anterior approach as it tends to rely more on intermuscular plane dissections which ultimately incites less microtrauma (13). This is reinforced by a study conducted by Bergin et al. which demonstrated lower levels of post-operative serum creatine kinase (CK) measurements in patients who underwent the anterior THA approach compared to that of its counterpart (14).

Lastly, the patient did not receive any prophylactic measures for prevention of heterotopic ossification during his hospitalization. Since the patient was previously healthy without predisposing risk factors and had a seemingly simple right posterior acetabular fracture-dislocation, it was reasonable that prophylactic treatments in the form of radiotherapy and/or non-steroidal anti-inflammatory drugs (NSAID) were not considered. However, it is known that NSAIDs and external beam radiation both act to reduce the incidence of ectopic ossification by suppressing the local inflammatory environment and inhibiting osteoblast differentiation within the osteogenic pathway. As such, prophylactic measures should be considered in critically ill patients with post-traumatic injuries as they are often inherently at higher risk of developing heterotopic ossifications.

Conclusion

In the case of our patient, the accelerated heterotopic ossification development is likely multifactorial. While the exact mechanism for such a rapid progression is largely speculative, factors which may have contributed include inflammation secondary to necrotizing pancreatitis, mechanical ventilation, immobility, delays in surgical intervention, surgical approach and the lack of prophylactic measures. In the future, it is valuable to consider early prophylactic measures in such critically ill patients given the elevated risk of pathological osseous development in this population.

Acknowledgments

We thank the generous support of Bratty Family Fund, Michael and Karyn Goldstein Cancer Research Fund, Joey and Mary Furfari Cancer Research Fund, Pulenzas Cancer Research Fund, Joseph and Silvana Melara Cancer Research Fund, and Ofelia Cancer Research Fund.

References

[1] McCarthy EF, Sundaram M. Heterotopic ossification: A review. Skeletal Radiol 2005;34(10):609-19.

[2] Gibon E, Lu L, Goodman SB. Aging, inflammation, stem cells, and bone healing. Stem Cell Res Ther 2016;7:44.

[3] Mavrogenis AF, Soucacos PN, Papagelopoulos PJ. Heterotopic ossification revisited. Orthopedics 2011;34(3):177.

[4] Jacobs JW, De Sonnaville PB, Hulsmans HM, van Rinsum AC, Bijlsma JW. Polyarticular heterotopic ossification complicating critical illness. Rheumatology (Oxford) 1999;38(11):1145-9.

[5] Herridge MS, Cheung AM, Tansey CM, Matte-Martyn A, Diaz-Granados N, Al-Saidi F, et al. One-year outcomes in survivors of the acute respiratory distress syndrome. N Engl J Med 2003;348(8):683-93.

[6] Shi S, de Gorter DJ, Hoogaars WM, Hoen PA, Dijke P. Overactive bone morphogenetic protein signaling in heterotopic ossification and Duchenne muscular dystrophy. Cell Mol Life Sci 2013;70(3):407-23.

[7] Glass GE, Chan JK, Freidin A, Feldmann M, Horwood NJ, Nanchahal J. TNF-alpha promotes fracture repair by augmenting the recruitment and differentiation of muscle-derived stromal cells. Proc Natl Acad Sci USA 2011;108(4):1585-90.

[8] Hudson SJ, Brett SJ. Heterotopic ossification-a long-term consequence of prolonged immobility. Crit Care 2006;10(6):174.

[9] Sugita A, Hashimoto J, Maeda A, Kobayashi J, Hirao M, Masuhara K, et al. Heterotopic ossification in bilateral knee and hip joints after long-term sedation. J Bone Miner Metab 2005;23(4):329-32.

[10] Pape HC, Lehmann U, van Griensven M, Gansslen A, von Glinski S, Krettek C. Heterotopic ossifications in patients after severe blunt trauma with and without head trauma: incidence and patterns of distribution. J Orthop Trauma 2001;15(4):229-37.

[11] Pape HC, Marsh S, Morley JR, Krettek C, Giannoudis PV. Current concepts in the development of heterotopic ossification. J Bone Joint Surg Br 2004;86(6):783-7.

[12] Wiggers JK, Helmerhorst GT, Brouwer KM, Niekel MC, Nunez F, Ring D. Injury complexity factors predict heterotopic ossification restricting motion after elbow trauma. Clin Orthop Relat Res 2014;472(7):2162-7.

[13] Newman EA, Holst DC, Bracey DN, Russell GB, Lang JE. Incidence of heterotopic ossification in direct anterior vs posterior approach to total hip arthroplasty: a retrospective radiographic review. Int Orthop 2016;40(9):1967-73.

[14] Bergin PF, Doppelt JD, Kephart CJ, Benke MT, Graeter JH, Holmes AS, et al. Comparison of minimally invasive direct anterior versus posterior total hip arthroplasty based on inflammation and muscle damage markers. J Bone Joint Surg Am 2011;93(15):1392-8.

In: Clinical Oncology
Editors: Ariel Tenenbaum et al.
ISBN: 978-1-53617-933-0

Chapter 9

ATYPICAL HEMANGIOMAS RESEMBLING METASTASES: A CASE REPORT AND REVIEW OF THE LITERATURE

Victoria Rico[1], Marjorie Monteiro Rodrigues[1], MD, Dominic Chan[1], Yasmeen Razvi[1], Erin McKenzie[1], Henry Lam[1], Carlo DeAngelis[1], PharmD, Edward Chow[1] and Fiona Lim[2,*]

[1]Sunnybrook Odette Cancer Centre, University of Toronto, Toronto, Ontario, Canada
[2]Princess Margaret Hospital, Hong Kong, PR China

* Corresponding Author: Fiona Lim, MDDS, Department of Clinical Oncology, Princess Margaret Hospital, Hong Kong, PRChina. E-mail: fionalimmy@gmail.com.

ABSTRACT

Hemangiomas of the bone account for 1% of all tumors found in the bone. Often asymptomatic in nature, many bone hemangiomas go undetected; however, when they are found on imaging, atypical-looking hemangiomas may be misdiagnosed as metastases in radiology. Methods: The present manuscript reports the case of a 50-year-old woman with a history of breast cancer presenting with a lesion at the T7 vertebra that was initially suspicious for a metastasis, but was later confirmed to be a vertebral bone hemangioma. A literature search with key words 'hemangioma' and 'metastases' was conducted on October 26, 2018 on Ovid Medline (1946 to October Week 2 2018) and Embase (1947 to 2018 week 43) to identify cases where bone hemangiomas were initially mistaken for bone metastases due to close resemblance. Results: Eighteen cases identified from the literature met the inclusion criteria for this review, in addition to the case from our centre as described above. The average age of patients included in this review was 56.7 years. Nine of 19 cases (47.4%) were prior to the diagnosis of bone hemangioma, while the remainder of the cases (n=10, 52.6%) reported symptoms which led to medical imaging and tests, and a final diagnosis of bone hemangioma. Relevant scans and tests, as well as follow-up information are described in detail. Conclusion: Determining optimal diagnostic methods and treatment protocols for bone hemangiomas should be a target for future investigation.

INTRODUCTION

Hemangiomas are benign vascular neoplasms composed of newly formed vessels or proliferated vessel walls and can occur anywhere in the human body (1). Bone hemangiomas represent 1% of all tumors found in the bone, and most commonly occur in the vertebrae and skull (2). There are four histological types of bone hemangiomas which include cavernous, capillary, arteriovenous, and venous (3). Hemangiomas arising in the bone are considered rare, however it is likely that many go undetected because of their slow growing and asymptomatic nature. Often, they are incidentally detected during radiographic examination of other lesions (1). In other cases, bone hemangiomas may produce symptoms, such as pain, visible or palpable alterations to the lesioned bone, and less commonly, osteomalacia, defined as delayed or defective mineralization of the bone, with bone fractures (4, 5) or spinal compression which may subsequently lead to neurological complications and deficits (6).

Undergoing staging evaluation is an essential step following a cancer diagnosis, as detecting or ruling out metastases based on these evaluations guides treatment plans and defines the intent of treatment for patients (7). In some cases however, benign entities, such as hemangiomas, may resemble metastases, potentially leading to unnecessary treatments including radiation therapy or chemotherapy (8).

Hemangiomas can usually be identified by their distinct appearance on radiography. Generally, hemangiomas have parallel line densities on x-ray due to their thickened vertical trabeculae (9, 10). Typical vertebral hemangioma appearances may be described as "corduroy cloth" due to the vertical striations; while a striated "honeycomb" or "sunburst" pattern is typical for hemangiomas of the skull (11). However, making a definitive diagnosis for bone hemangiomas can be difficult when they appear as atypical. Features found on magnetic resonance imaging (MRI) are largely impacted by the amount of vascularity and fat that compose the lesions. Areas of high signal intensity in T1-weighted MRI are due to high-fat content, and areas of high signal intensity in T2-weighted MRI are due to vascularity of lesions (12). Typical hemangiomas show high-intensity on T1 and T2-weighted images on MRI, as well as coarsened vertical trabeculae on computed tomography (CT) and radiographic imaging (13). On axial CT scans, hemangiomas of the spine would appear as having a "polkadot" pattern (14). Further, CT scans of hemangiomas in the metaphysis and epiphysis of the long bones typically appear as lytic lesions with spiculated pattern (14). Atypical hemangiomas appear hypointense on T1-weighted MRI but have the typical characteristics usually seen in T2-weighted images (15). This atypical appearance may look like a metastatic lesion which usually has low T1-weighted signals, while having high T2-weighted signals on MRI (16). On bone scintigraphy, bone hemangiomas may appear as photopenic and they may also have a moderate increase in radiotracer uptake (17).

The present manuscript describes a patient treated at our centre for breast cancer with an identified lesion at T7 that was suspicious for a metastasis. Upon further investigation the lesion was favoured to be a bone hemangioma. All available literature on bone hemangiomas resembling metastases or being misdiagnosed as metastases are systematically reviewed below (3, 10, 22–27, 11, 14, 15, 17–21). To our knowledge, this is the first literature review of its kind. This review aims to examine commonalities between these atypical hemangiomas, as well as imaging techniques that may be used to aid in a more accurate diagnosis of hemangiomas.

CASE REPORT

A 50-year-old perimenopausal woman presented with self-detected right breast mass with occasional pain and burning sensation at the site of the mass. A right breast ultrasound revealed an irregular solid 2.6 cm mass, suspicious for malignancy, with a Breast Imaging Reporting and Data System (BI-RADS) score of 4. She then had a bilateral mammogram which revealed a 3.2 cm mass in the upper-outer right breast at the site of the questioned palpable lump. A second bilateral mammogram revealed a 3.3 cm spiculated mass in the upper outer right breast with prominent lymph nodes anterior to the mass. A 0.5 cm obscured mass medial to the dominant mass was also observed.

The patient underwent an ultrasound guided biopsy of the index lesion, and pathological analysis revealed a well-differentiated invasive ductal carcinoma with no lymphovascular invasion (LVI). The biomarkers were estrogen receptor (ER) and progesterone receptor (PR) positive, and human epidermal growth factor receptor 2 (HER2) negative.

She underwent a right-sided, skin-sparing, simple mastectomy with sentinel lymph node biopsy (SLNB) and immediate reconstruction with a deep inferior epigastric perforators flap. The mastectomy specimen revealed 11 foci of multifocal invasive ductal carcinoma, with the largest foci being 3.5 cm. The specimen was of low grade with a minor DCIS component. The margins of the invasive carcinoma and the DCIS were clear. Two intramammary lymph nodes were positive with macrometastasis, one of which contained extranodal extension, and one sentinel lymph node was positive with macrometastasis with extranodal capsular involvement.

The patient then began dose-dense adjuvant chemotherapy regimen consisting of Doxorubicin, Cyclophosphamide for initial four cycles and Paclitaxel for latter four cycles (AC-Pacli) given intravenously once every two weeks for a total of eight treatments.

Staging evaluations including a chest, abdomen, and pelvis CT scans, and bone scan to ensure that there was no distant spread of her disease were performed. The chest CT revealed a well-defined hypodense lesion within the right aspect of the T7 vertebral body measuring 10 mm and was suspicious for metastases. Subsequent MRI showed focal hemangiomas within the spinal vertebrae at T1, T2, T4-T5, T6, T9, T12 and L2 levels, and degenerative changes at multiple levels of the cervical and lumbar spine, with no evidence of vertebral expansion, collapseor significant bony encroachment of the spinal canal or perivertebral soft tissue thickening. The focal lucent area within the T7 vertebral body on the right side showed mild T2 hyperintensity with a peripheral low signal intensity rim and isointense on the T1-weighted image. These findings of the T7 lesion were indeterminate, although its morphology favoured a more benign etiology.

She was then referred to a specialized bone metastases clinic to be seen by a radiation oncologist and an orthopaedic surgeon for further investigation of the suspicious T7 lesion. Upon further review of the imaging of the lesion, it was favoured to be a benign bone hemangioma and not metastases. The patient reported some concern about a recent onset of mild discomfort in her lower back and neck, which was suggestive to be degenerative spine disease, or secondary to her chemotherapy and granulocyte-colony stimulating factor injection.

The patient was reassured, and observation and follow-up imaging in three months was recommended. The patient continued with her chemotherapy, and at follow-up one month later was doing well with no symptoms related to her bone hemangiomas.

LITERATURE REVIEW

A literature search was conducted on October 26, 2018 on Ovid Medline (1946 to October Week 2 2018) and Embase (1947 to 2018 week 43). The keywords that were used in this search included 'hemangioma' and 'metastases.' The searches were limited to English language and human subjects only.

Data extraction

Articles were first screened by title and abstract independently by two authors (VR and YR). Potential articles for inclusion were subsequently full-text screened independently by two authors (VR and MMR). A complete description of the screening process can be found in Figure 1.

Articles met the inclusion criteria for this review if they described cases that reported on hemangiomas of the bone or where an incorrect diagnosis or speculation of metastases instead of hemangioma was originally made. The exclusion criteria for this review included: i) hemangiomas located in places other than the bone, ii) hemangiomas where potential metastasis was not considered during the diagnostic process, iii) articles that did not report information on individual cases. Non-original articles, including reviews and editorials were also excluded.

Available information on patient characteristics, medical histories, hemangioma characteristics, scan or test results, medications, treatments, and follow-up outcomes were extracted by two authors (VR and MMR) and can be found in Table 1.

Table 1. Patient characteristics, scan findings, and follow-ups

Author (year)	Age	Sex (M/F)	Cancer type (stage)	Site of bone heman-gioma	Size of heman-gioma (cm)	Symptoms that led to dx	Relevant scan/test findings	Tx for hemangioma	Medical history	Medications	FU, number of months	Histolo-gical subtype
Park, et al. [(18)]	63	M	None	L 6th rib	5.5 x 2.5 x 1.5	None	**CT**: Osteolytic eccentric expansive mass w/ sunburst calcification and focal cortical disruption at posterolateral arc of L 6th rib; 18F-FDG PET/CT: lesion showed SUV max of 2.4 **Histopathologic analysis of rib**: thin-walled blood vessels w/ dilated channels w/ red blood cells, lined by layer of endothelial cells	Rib resection via postlateral thoracotomy approach	Hypertension	Anti-hypertensive medication (NS)	x	Cavernous
Raphael, et al. [(3)] (case 1)	46	F	Cervix (I)	L1 vertebra	x	Back pain	**Bone scan**: increased tracer uptake in L1 vertebra; **SPECT-CT:** increased tracer uptake in L1 vertebral body;	x	x	x	FOD, 6	x

Table 1. (Continued)

Author (year)	Age	Sex (M/F)	Cancer type (stage)	Site of bone heman-gioma	Size of heman-gioma (cm)	Symptoms that led to dx	Relevant scan/test findings	Tx for hemangioma	Medical history	Medications	FU, number of months	Histolo-gical subtype
							MRI: well-defined lesion, hyperintense on T1 and T2-weighted images, multi hypointense dots within T2-weighted images; **PET-CT:** no evidence of increased metabolic activity in L1 vertebra lesion, and osteolytic area at L1					
Raphael, et al. [(3)] (case 2)	54	F	Breast	Multiple vertebral and rib heman-giomas	x	x	**Bone scan**: abnormal increase in tracer uptake in L 2nd rib and thoracolumbar vertebrae; **CT thorax**: multiple hemangiomas of the vertebrae and ribs; **PET-CT**: ruled out skeletal metastases	x	x	x	FOD, 24	x

Author (year)	Age	Sex (M/F)	Cancer type (stage)	Site of bone heman-gioma	Size of heman-gioma (cm)	Symptoms that led to dx	Relevant scan/test findings	Tx for hemangioma	Medical history	Medications	FU, number of months	Histolo-gical subtype
Manohar, et al. [(19)]	64	M	Renal cell	D8, L4, D10, L3 vertebrae	x	x	**Bone scintigraphy with MDP:** increased tracer uptake in D8, L4 vertebrae; **SPECT/CT:** MDP uptake in D8 was localized to hemangioma with vertical trabecular thickening on CT, L4 showed MDP avidity with intralesional trabecular thickening, similar lesions seen in D10 and L3 vertebrae; **FDG PET/CT:** no FDG uptake in the lesions, ruling out metastasis	x	x	x	x	x
Daoud, et al. [(10)]	56	F	None	Cervical, thoracic, and lumbar vertebrae, lower sternum, L ischial bone, R iliac crest, L posterior 6th rib,	x	Chronic lower back and neck pain	**Lumbo-sacral X-ray**: osteoblastic lesions in lumbar vertebrae, R iliac crest, and L sacro-iliac joint; **CT pelvis**: areas of increased bone density with surrounding cortical bone destruction in L ischial bone, R iliac crest and	Analgesics	Bronchial asthma, microscopic hematuria, osteoporosis	Calcium supplements, alendronate	Doing well, pain free, no new lesions, 12	x

Table 1. (Continued)

Author (year)	Age	Sex (M/F)	Cancer type (stage)	Site of bone heman-gioma	Size of heman-gioma (cm)	Symptoms that led to dx	Relevant scan/test findings	Tx for hemangioma	Medical history	Medications	FU, number of months	Histolo-gical subtype
				R femoral bone			L sacro-iliac joint suggesting osteoblastic metastasis; **Tc whole body scan:** multiple bony lesions in cervical, thoracic and lumbar vertebra, lower sternum, L ischial bone, R iliac crest, L posterior 6th rib, R femoral bone suggesting bone metastases; **L pelvic bone biopsy**: sclerosing type of bone hemangioma					
Usmani, et al. [(17)]	66	M	Prostate	D4 vertebra	x	x	**PET-CT:** solitary osteoblastic lesion at D4 vertebral body; **MRI:** features of atypical hemangioma; **Ga-68 PSMA PET-CT:** no signs of bone metastasis;	x	x	x	x	x

Author (year)	Age	Sex (M/F)	Cancer type (stage)	Site of bone hemangioma	Size of hemangioma (cm)	Symptoms that led to dx	Relevant scan/test findings	Tx for hemangioma	Medical history	Medications	FU, number of months	Histological subtype
							^{18}F-naF PET-CT (8-month FU): persistent osteoblastic lesion at D4 without significant change, confirming atypical hemangioma					
Dang et al. [(20)]	41	F	None	Vertebral body, L pedicles, and lamina of L5, spinal canal, paravertebral region	x	Intermittent back pain for 18 months; numbness of L thoracic wall with intermittent radiating pain; tenderness along middle thoracic spine	**CT:** osteolytic lesion in vertebral body, L pedicles, T5 lamina, disrupted T5 cortex **MRI:** tumor invading entirety of T5 vertebral body, spinal canal and paravertebral region, heterogeneously hypointense on T1-weighted image and hyperintense on T2-weighted image, significant increase in signal intensity; **MRI:** compression of dural sac by epidural extension of tumor; **PET-CT:** T5 lesion, SUV of 1.3 Biopsy of paravertebral lesion:	Combined laminectomy + vertebroplasty; excision of the epidural soft tumor mass; postoperative RT 30Gy 4 weeks after surgery	x	x	x	x

Table 1. (Continued)

Author (year)	Age	Sex (M/F)	Cancer type (stage)	Site of bone hemangioma	Size of hemangioma (cm)	Symptoms that led to dx	Relevant scan/test findings	Tx for hemangioma	Medical history	Medications	FU, number of months	Histological subtype
							distinct histopathological diagnosis of vertebral hemangioma					
Shi et al. [(21)]	60	F	None	Tll vertebra	x	x	Isointense signal lesion at T11-vertebrae on T1-weighted image; isointense signal of fat suppressed T1-weighted images; **CT:** hypo-dense lesion with internal striated appearance	x	x	x	x	
Ching et al. [(14)]	52	F	None	L knee	x	L lower limb pain for several years; L knee pain leading to impaired mobility; weight loss	**Radiograph:** isodense lesion to the bone located within the medullary cavity, with a sclerotic margin at epiphysis of proximal tibia and lesion with central lucency with a sclerotic margin at the diaphysis of L femur and proximal L fibula;	Open biopsy w/segmental osteotomy	Stage I membranous nephropathy; hypertension	Yes / treated symptomatically (NS)	Pain free, 12	Mixed capillary and venous

Author (year)	Age	Sex (M/F)	Cancer type (stage)	Site of bone heman-gioma	Size of heman-gioma (cm)	Symptoms that led to dx	Relevant scan/test findings	Tx for hemangioma	Medical history	Medications	FU, number of months	Histolo-gical subtype
							Surgical biopsy w/ osteotomy of L mid fibula: thin-walled blood vessels w/ adjacent bony trabeculae, vascular channels of dilated venous-calibre type and capillary sized vessels, no malignant cells					
Lakemeier, et al. [(22)]	44	F	None	C7 vertebra	x	Paresthesia in forearms + hands for 3 months; pain + paresthesia in face	**X-ray:** osteolysis of C7 vertebra; **MRI:** increased signal intensity on T2-weighted images, diagnosis of metastatic osteolysis of C7 was made; **Intensive immuno-histochemical work-up:** distinct vascularization of lesion with partially collapsed sinusoidal and slit-like blood vessels, no cytologic atypia or increased mitotic rate were seen,	Corporectomy of C7; implantation of customary titanium cage	None	x	Pain free cervical spine movement, loss of rotation of 20 degrees, normal alignment of spine, 6	Capillary

Table 1. (Continued)

Author (year)	**Age**	**Sex (M/F)**	**Cancer type (stage)**	**Site of bone heman-gioma**	**Size of heman-gioma (cm)**	**Symptoms that led to dx**	**Relevant scan/test findings**	**Tx for hemangioma**	**Medical history**	**Medications**	**FU, number of months**	**Histolo-gical subtype**
							hemangioma with reactive osteoid formation was made					
Wallis et al. [(23)]	52	F	None	Iliac crest; dorsal and lumbo-sacral spine; ribs; skull	x	7 year history of dull, sharp, shooting back pain, radiating in a bilateral radicular distribution, around lower thorax, abdomen, and hips, thighs, knees, legs and ankles	**Roentgenograms of chest:** extensive metastases in the lungs, osteoblastic and osteolytic metastases in the skull, pelvis, spine, and long bones, lytic lesions in both ilia; **Thyroidectomy:** nodular goiter and no evidence of carcinoma, ruling out the thyroid as the primary source of metastases; **Lung biopsy:** nodular fibrosis of unknown etiology; **Rib biopsy:** normal bone and skeletal muscle;	1000 calorie diet; exercise regimen; thyroid replacement; dextropropoxyphene; 2700 cGy to lumbar spine	Hemorrhoids caused by constipation, chronic cigarette cough, obesity, hard nodule on thyroid	x	Mild occasional backaches, NS	Mixed capillary and cavernous

Author (year)	Age	Sex (M/F)	Cancer type (stage)	Site of bone heman-gioma	Size of heman-gioma (cm)	Symptoms that led to dx	Relevant scan/test findings	Tx for hemangioma	Medical history	Medications	FU, number of months	Histolo-gical subtype
							Iliac biopsy: mixed capillary and cavernous hemangioma of the bone					
Leeds et al. [(15)]	40	x	Ocular melanoma; hepatic metastasis	L2 vertebral body	x	x	**MRI:** abnormal increase in sagittal T1-weighted signal intensity of lesion, decrease in signal intensity on sagittal FSE T2-weighted, fat-suppressed image, intense enhancement on postcontrast sagittal T1 weighted, fat-suppressed image; **CT:** A sharply defined lesion with trabecular pattern	x	x	x	x	x
Leeds et al. [(15)]	x	x	x	L3 vertebral body	x	x	**MRI:** A sharply defined lesion with low signal intensity on T1-weighted image, high signal intensity on T2 with fat suppression and homogeneous intense enhancement on post-contrast sagittal T1	x	x	x	x	x

Table 1. (Continued)

Author (year)	Age	Sex (M/F)	Cancer type (stage)	Site of bone heman-gioma	Size of heman-gioma (cm)	Symptoms that led to dx	Relevant scan/test findings	Tx for hemangioma	Medical history	Medications	FU, number of months	Histolo-gical subtype
							fat-suppressed image; **Axial post-contrast T1-weighted MRI:** prominent basivertebral plexus, draining from the hemangioma, distinct vascular channel					
Laguna et al. [(24)]	62	M	Papillary thyroid carcinoma with metastases to cervical nodes	T5 vertebra	x	None	**Whole-body I-131 scan**: abnormal focal area of I-131 tracer concentration in the chest; **CT spine:** dense trabecular pattern in the vertebral body resembling a hemangioma	x	x	x	Symptom free, NS	x
Zito et al.[(11)]	58	M	x	Skull, T2, T3, T6, T9, T10, L4, T6, sacrum	x	Bilateral leg weakness; difficulty walking; occasional falls; burning pain in the back and	**X-ray of spine and pelvis:** lucent areas with parallel vertical striations in T2, T3, T6, T9, T10, L4, and L5 bodies, similar lesion in the R superior sacrum,	Intravenous dexamethasone therapy, and a decompressive laminectomy was performed from T2 to T6	x	Intravenous dexamethasone therapy, decompressive laminectomy from T2 to T6	No neurological abnormalities except mild proximal leg weakness and hyperreflexia	Capillary

Author (year)	Age	Sex (M/F)	Cancer type (stage)	Site of bone heman-gioma	Size of heman-gioma (cm)	Symptoms that led to dx	Relevant scan/test findings	Tx for hemangioma	Medical history	Medications	FU, number of months	Histolo-gical subtype
						legs; a band-like sensation around the mid-thorax; urinary urgency; incomplete bladder emptying; constipation	paravertebral mass in the midthoracic region, oval radiolucent lesion in the L frontal bone w/ honeycomb like appearance; **Myelography:** compressive lesion blocking upward flow at T6 and downward flow at T2; **Spinal angiography:** vascular lesions at T6 & T10, w/ prominent extraosseous staining; **Biopsy of T2 vertebrae:** capillary hemangioma					
Kulshrestha et al. [(25)]	45	M	None	T1 vertebra; R 9th rib; L 8th rib	x	Coldness, numbness and clumsiness in the legs; exacerbated by neck flexion or hand use, which caused "pins	**Thyroid scan:** increased uptake in one lobe, appearing to be a benign adenoma; **Bone scan**: increased uptake at T1, R 9th rib, 10th rib; **MRI:** increase in signal intensity on T2 weighted images, as well as mottled	Vertebrectomy for neural decompression (prior to hemangioma diagnosis); embolization therapy via a branch of T5 intercostal artery	Appendec-tomy; spontaneous pneumo-thorax	x	Symptom-free	x

Table 1. (Continued)

Author (year)	Age	Sex (M/F)	Cancer type (stage)	Site of bone heman-gioma	Size of heman-gioma (cm)	Symptoms that led to dx	Relevant scan/test findings	Tx for hemangioma	Medical history	Medications	FU, number of months	Histolo-gical subtype
						and needles" or electric shocks to go down the backs of his legs to the soles of his feet	appearance of T1 vertebral body. This was reported as metastatic disease; **Vertebrectomy:** when attempted, caused massive arterial bleeding from the bone, thus only partial removal of T1 body was possible; **Histopathological analysis of bone removed from vertebrectomy:** wide thin-walled blood-filled spaces and sinuses lined by endothelium interspersed among trabeculae of bone, typical of bone hemangioma; **CT of T1:** revealed vertebral hemangioma;					

Author (year)	Age	Sex (M/F)	Cancer type (stage)	Site of bone heman-gioma	Size of heman-gioma (cm)	Symptoms that led to dx	Relevant scan/test findings	Tx for hemangioma	Medical history	Medications	FU, number of months	Histolo-gical subtype
							CT of L 8th and R 9th ribs: vertical trabeculae, consistent with bone hemangioma					
Puri et al. [(26)]	63	M	None	4th rib	6.5x5x2.5	L chest wall pain; dyspnea	**X-ray chest:** radiopaque shadow in L mid and lower zone; **Contrast enhanced CT:** heterogenous, expansile, osteolytic, eccentric bony outgrowth at 4th rib; histopathological examination of rib: encapsulated, globular, expansible lesion which measured 6.5x5x2.5 cm in size, cut surface showed cystic degeneration filled with hemorrhage, dilated and congested thin and thick-walled vascular spaces, bony trabeculae lined by conspicuous	x	x	x	x	x

Table 1. (Continued)

Author (year)	Age	Sex (M/F)	Cancer type (stage)	Site of bone heman-gioma	Size of heman-gioma (cm)	Symptoms that led to dx	Relevant scan/test findings	Tx for hemangioma	Medical history	Medications	FU, number of months	Histolo-gical subtype
							osteoblastic rimming present, diagnosed as hemangioma					
Bellasri et al. [(27)]	40	F	None	T7 vertebrae		Dorsal pain; weakness and numbness in lower limbs; Upgoing toes bilaterally; bilateral patellar tendon hyperreflexia	**MRI:** T7 expansile bone mass involving spine, low T1 signal intensity, heterogeneous high T2 signal intensity; **Surgery with posterior approach:** highly vascularized lesion; **Histologic analysis:** numerous think walled vascular channels in collagenous connective tissue, with single layer of endothelial cells, hemangioma diagnosis made	Complete resection of tumor	x	x	No pain or weakness; walking with normal posture; significant spinal cord decompression, 1-week post-op; 4 weeks; 2 months	Cavernous

Author (year)	Age	Sex (M/F)	Cancer type (stage)	Site of bone heman-gioma	Size of heman-gioma (cm)	Symptoms that led to dx	Relevant scan/test findings	Tx for hemangioma	Medical history	Medications	FU, number of months	Histolo-gical subtype
Rico et al. (present case)	50	F	Breast	T1, T2, T4, T5, T6, T7, T9, T12, L2 vertebrae	T7: 10mm	None	**Chest CT:** well-defined hypodensity with R aspect of T7 vertebral body; **MRI:** focal hemangiomas within spinal vertebrae at T1, T2, T4, T5, T6, T9, T12, L2	None	x	x	Symptom free, 1	x

M, male; F, female; Tx, treatment; SUV max, maximum standardized uptake value; CT, Computed Tomography; NS, not specified; BS, bone scan; RT, radiation therapy; MDP, methylene diphosphate; FDG, fluorodeoxyglucose; PET, positron emission tomography; SPECT, single photon emission computed tomography; L, left; R, right; Mets, metastasis; MRI, magnetic resonance imaging; Ga-68 PSMA, Gallium-68-prostate-specific membrane antigen; 18F-naF PET-CT, 18F-sodium fluoride positron emission tomography-computed tomography; FOD, free of disease; NS, not specified.

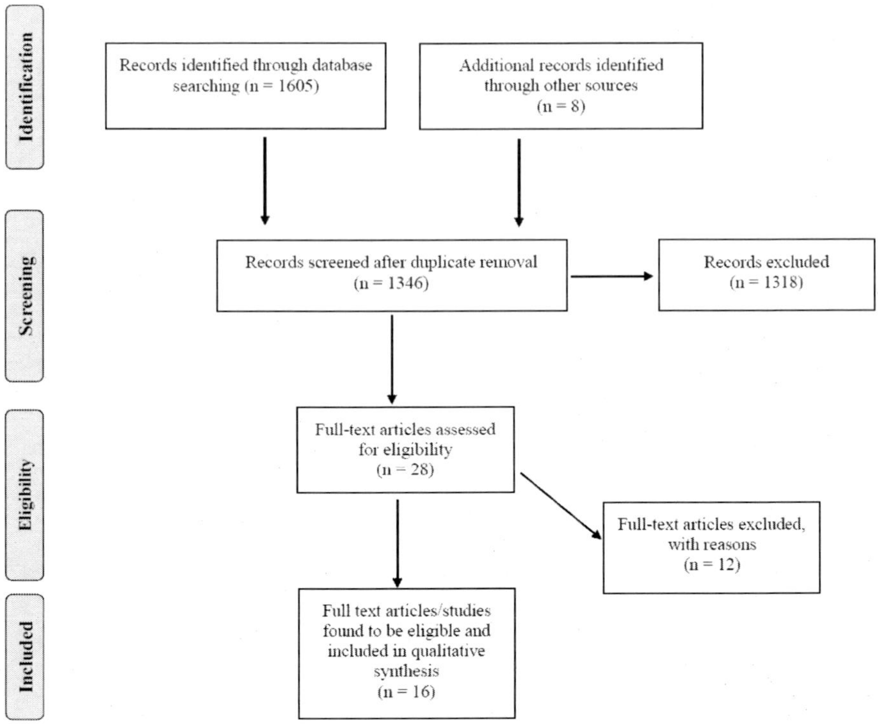

Figure 1. Flowchart of article screening and selection process.

SEARCH RESULTS

The literature search generated a total of 1,605 articles: 1,210 from Embase, and 395 from Ovid Medline. A total of 24 articles were included for full text screening. Of the 24 articles that were full-text screened, 16 articles met the inclusion criteria for this review (3, 8-22). Table 1 contains a summary of the reviewed articles, including patient characteristics, relevant scans and tests and patient-reported symptoms.

Patient characteristics

This literature review summarizes 19 cases of bone hemangiomas that resembled or were initially misdiagnosed as bone metastases (3, 8-22). Eighteen of 19 cases reported age, and the average age across these 18 cases was 56.6 years and ranged from 40 to 66 years old. Sex was reported in 17 of 19 cases (89.5%), with 7 of 17 cases being male patients (41.2%), and 10 of 17 cases being female patients (58.8%) (3, 8, 10-22).

In 12 of 19 cases (63.2%), it was stated that the patient either did not have cancer, or there was no primary cancer reported; thus, we assumed that they did not have cancer (10, 11, 14, 15, 18, 20–23, 25-27). Among the seven patients that reported a primary cancer, the most common site was the breast (n=2, 10.5%).

Ten of 19 hemangioma cases (52.6%) occurred solely in the spinal or vertebral region, and five cases (26.3%) featured multiple hemangiomas of the spinal or vertebral region, in addition to other bony sites; thus, 15 of 19 cases (79.0%) had vertebral or spinal hemangiomas (3, 11, 15, 17, 19–27). Two of 19 cases (10.5%) reported on hemangiomas occurring in the rib alone, while four cases (21.1%) reported on rib hemangiomas in addition to hemangiomas in other bone regions; thus, a total of six cases reported on hemangiomas of the rib (31.6%) (3, 10, 18, 23, 25, 26). Two cases reported on hemangiomas of the skull in addition to other bone regions (10.5%) (11, 23). Other regions that bone hemangiomas were found are summarized in Table 1.

Nine of 19 cases (47.4%) either reported that the patient had no symptoms associated with the bone hemangioma, or no symptoms were described; thus, we assumed they were asymptomatic (3, 15, 17–19, 21, 24). Ten of 19 patients (52.6%) reported at least one symptom, such as back pain (n=5, 50.0%) or leg weakness and numbness (n=3, 30.0%) in patients presenting with vertebral hemangiomas (3, 10, 11, 14, 20, 22, 23, 25, 27). One patient (10.0%) with a rib hemangioma reported chest wall pain (26). One patient (10.0%) with a cervical vertebral hemangioma reported paresthesia in her forearms and hands, as well as pain and paresthesia in her face (22). Another patient (10.0%) with a knee hemangioma reported pain in her lower limb and knee area (14). Additional symptoms reported by patients are described in Table 1.

Nine of 19 patients (47.4%) underwent some type of treatment or intervention for their bone hemangioma (3, 10, 11, 14, 15, 17–21, 23-27) described in greater detail in Table 1. Of note, not all patients who received intervention presented with symptoms, as some of these interventions were done to aid in the diagnosis of the bone hemangioma, rather than treat symptoms associated with the hemangioma.

Histological subtype data was only available for five of 19 patients (26.3%) (14, 18, 22, 27, 28). Of these five patients, two were cavernous (40.0%) (18, 27), one was capillary (20.0%) (22), one was mixed capillary and cavernous (20.0%) (23), and one was mixed capillary and venous (20.0%) (14).

Follow-up information was available for 11 of 19 patients (57.9%) (3, 10, 11, 14, 22–25, 27). Two of 19 (10.5%) patients were free-of-disease at follow-up (3). Seven of 19 patients (36.8%) were symptom or pain-free at follow-up (10, 14, 22, 24, 25, 27). One patient (5.3%) reported mild, occasional back pain at follow-up (23). One patient (5.3%) reported no neurological abnormalities but had proximal leg weakness and hyperreflexia at follow–up (11).

DISCUSSION

Diagnosing bone hemangiomas can be difficult when they appear as atypical upon medical imaging. Bone hemangiomas that are mistakenly diagnosed as bone metastases can lead to additional anxiety and worry for patients and family members and non-essential tests and imaging (29). Determining effective diagnostic strategies to differentiate hemangiomas and metastases should be a target for future investigation. Additionally, determining treatment protocol and management of bone hemangiomas should be a focus of study in the future.

Bone hemangiomas are rare, and most commonly occur in the vertebrae and skull (2). Large autopsy studies and radiographic scan reviews have concluded that hemangiomas are the most common benign lesions found in the spine, with an approximate incidence of 10-12% within the general population (30). After reviewing the literature, 15 of 19 cases (79.0%) involved vertebral or spinal hemangiomas mistaken for metastases; while only two of 19 cases (10.5%) involved hemangiomas of the skull mistaken for metastases. This may suggest that despite being a common type of hemangioma, skull hemangiomas may present with a more typical appearance on radiographic imaging than vertebral hemangiomas, resulting in less frequent confusion with metastases.

When hemangiomas appear as atypical, many of the classic characteristics of hemangiomas that aid in their diagnosis are not present (14). MRI is regarded as the imaging modality that provides the clearest description of hemangiomas (10). However, MRI intensities of atypical hemangiomas may not lead to a direct diagnosis of hemangioma, and thus, examining the morphology of the lesion may help aid in making an accurate diagnosis. CT scans may be used in these cases, since they have a higher sensitivity for detecting bone remodeling (17). While diagnosis of bone hemangiomas is frequently accomplished based on radiographic appearance of the hemangioma, in atypical hemangioma cases a bone biopsy is warranted to differentiate from metastasis, cysts or other bony lesions (31). To illustrate the challenges with atypical hemangiomas, Ching et al. noted that typical hemangiomas of non-spinal sites are radiolucent, expansile and are distinct with a radiating type pattern; however, one of their hemangioma cases was found to have both lucent and isodense areas, with reactive sclerotic margins, suggestive of osteoid osteoma (14). Moreover, Ching et al. (14) described another case where on CT scan, a vertebral hemangioma appeared to have ring-shaped lucencies with sclerotic rings, which differs from the typical polka-dot appearance of vertebral body hemangiomas (14).

Bone hemangiomas are often found incidentally on scanning assessments due to their asymptomatic tendencies. Including the reviewed cases and the case from our centre, nine of 19 cases (47.4%) had no reported symptoms associated with their bone hemangioma (3, 15, 17–19, 21, 24). It is important to note that symptomatic patients may have been experiencing such symptoms as a result of their cancer, and not necessarily because of the hemangioma itself. A study that examined 59 cases of vertebral hemangiomas from 1980 to 1990 found 35 (59.3%) of these hemangiomas incidentally, and 13 of them (22.0%) due to associated pain. This study highlighted the asymptomatic nature of bone hemangiomas and noted that they are often found incidentally.

Given that hemangiomas are often asymptomatic in nature, they commonly do not require medical intervention or treatment. However, in cases where hemangiomas are more aggressive, they may require treatment. Although rare, some vertebral hemangiomas may act aggressively and invade the paravertebral space or spinal canal, resulting in potential compression of the spinal cord or nerve roots (30). Occurrence of such compressions are seen most commonly in hemangiomas of the thoracic spine (30). There is no clear consensus among health care providers on the standard treatment protocol for aggressive hemangiomas and thus, these concepts should be further explored.

Fox et al. (30) historically reviewed 11 patients with vertebral hemangiomas with spinal cord compression. All 11 patients initially underwent decompressive surgery and had complete neurological recovery. Six patients underwent subtotal tumor resection and subsequent radiation therapy (RT) of 1000 cGy or less; of which three patients (50.0%) had recurrent neurological symptoms. All four patients who underwent subtotal tumor resection plus RT had no recurrences. One patient who underwent gross tumor resection did not recur when examined at follow-up of an unspecified time period. These patient findings and a review of the literature led the authors of this article to recommend yearly neurological and radiological examination in patients with painful hemangiomas, and stated that this is particularly important for young females with thoracic hemangiomas. RT and embolization are also effective treatments for individuals with moderate to severe constant pain. The authors state that those with asymptomatic hemangiomas do not require regular follow-up, unless pain corresponding to the hemangioma develops. The authors conclude that patients with neurological deficits should undergo preoperative embolization and angiography, decompressive surgery, and RT in patients who undergo subtotal tumor resection (30).

Uncertainty surrounding imaging methods for bone hemangiomas remain a clinical challenge and determining the best detection methods for these lesions should be the focus of future investigation. Forming a consensus for treatment protocols of bone hemangiomas should be another target for studies. Bone hemangiomas, especially those that are atypical in appearance, may lead to diagnostic and treatment uncertainty. In such cases where lesions are equivocal or indeterminate, a radiologist should be consulted to proceed with a diagnosis and treatment plan.

ACKNOWLEDGMENTS

We thank the generous support of Bratty Family Fund, Michael and Karyn Goldstein Cancer Research Fund, Joey and Mary Furfari Cancer Research Fund, Pulenzas Cancer Research Fund, Joseph and Silvana Melara Cancer Research Fund, and Ofelia Cancer Research Fund. The authors declare that there is no conflict of interest. Written consent was obtained from the patient to allow for the publication of this report and any relevant accompanying images.

REFERENCES

[1] Pack GT, Miller TR. Hemangiomas: Classification, diagnosis and treatment. Angiology 1950;1(5):405–26.

[2] Dorfman HD, Steinel GC, Jaffe HL. Vascular tumors of the bone. Hum Pathol 1971;2(3):349–76.

[3] Raphael J, Hephzibah J, Mani S, Shanthly N, Oommen R. Abnormal appearance of spinal hemangioma mimicking metastasis in bone scintigraphy and SPECT-CT: Case report. J Nucl Med Radiat Ther 2013;S6(016):1–3.

[4] Rokan Z, Kealey WD. Osteomalacia: A forgotten cause of fractures in the elderly. BMJ Case Rep 2015;2015:1–2. doi: 10.1136/bcr-2014-207184.

[5] McCarthy EF, Frassica FJ. Pathology of bone and joint disorders with clinical and radiographic correlation. Cambridge: Cambridge University Press, 2014.

[6] Aksu G, Fayda M, Saynak M, Karadeniz A. Spinal cord compression due to vertebral hemangioma. Orthopedics 2008;31(2):169.

[7] Heindel W, Gübitz R, Vieth V, Weckesser M, Schober O, Schäfers M. The diagnostic imaging of bone metastases. Dtsch Arztebl Int 2014;111(44):741–7.

[8] Morales KA, Arevalo-Perez J, Holodny AI, Lis E, Karimi S. Differentiating atypical hemangiomas and metastatic vertebral lesions? The role of T1-weighted dynamic. Am Soc Neuroradiol 2018;39(5):968-73.

[9] Rodallec MH, Feydy A, Larousserie F, Anract P, Campagna R, Babinet A, et al. Diagnostic imaging of solitary tumors of the spine: What to do and say. Radiographics 2008;28(4):1019–41.

[10] Daoud E. Multiple bone hemangiomas presenting as bony metastasis of unknown primary. J Med 2010;11(2):196–9.

[11] Zito G, Kadis GN. Multiple vertebral hemangiomas resembling metastases with spinal cord compression. Arch Neurol 1980;37(4):247–8.

[12] Ross JS, Masaryk TJ, Modic MT, Carter JR, Mapstone T, Dengel FH. Vertebral hemangiomas: MR imaging. Radiology 1987;165(1):165–9.

[13] Gaudino S, Martucci M, Colantonio R, Lozupone E, Visconti E, Leone A, et al. A systematic approach to vertebral hemangioma. Skeletal Radiol 2015;44(1):25–36.

[14] Ching BC, Wong JSL, Tan MH, Jara-lazaro AR. The many faces of intraosseous haemangioma: A diagnostic headache. Singapore Med J 2009;50(5):195–8.

[15] Leeds NE, Kumar A, Zhou XJ, McKinnon GC. Magnetic resonance imaging of benign spinal lesions simulating metastasis: Role of diffusion-weighted imaging. Top Magn Reson Imaging 2000;11(4):224–34.

[16] Cross JJ, Antoun NM, Laing RJC, Xuereb J. Imaging of compressive vertebral haemangiomas. Eur Radiol 2000;10(6):997–1002.

[17] Usmani S, Marafi F, Rasheed R, Al Kandari F, Ahmed N. Atypical hemangioma mimicking metastasis on 18F-sodium fluoride positron emission tomography-computed tomography and magnetic resonance imaging: Gallium-68-prostate-specific membrane antigen positron emission tompgraphy improves the specificity of bone lesions. Indian J Nucl Med 2018;33(2):171–3.

[18] Park JY, Gyoon PJ, Lee SJ. Cavernous hemangioma of the breast: A case report. Iran J Radiol 2016;13(3):1–3.

[19] Manohar K, Paraghane R, Kumari S, Bhattacharya A, Mandal A, Mittal B. Multiple vertebral hemangiomas mimicking metastases in a patient with renal carcinoma: Importance of hybrid imaging with SPECT/CT and FDG PET/CT. J Postgrad Med 2012;46(4):196–7.

[20] Dang L, Liu C, Yang SM, Jiang L, Liu ZJ, Liu XG, et al. Aggressive vertebral hemangioma of the thoracic spine without typical radiological appearance. Eur Spine J 2012;21(10):1994–9.

[21] Shi Y-J, Li X-T, Zhang X-Y, Liu Y-L, Tang L, Sun Y-S. Differential diagnosis of hemangiomas from spinal osteolytic metastases using 3.0 T MRI: Comparison of T1-weighted imaging, chemical-shift imaging, diffusion-weighted and contrast-enhanced imaging. Oncotarget 2017;8(41):71095–104.

[22] Lakemeier S, Westhoff CC, Fuchs-Winkelmann S, Schofer MD. Osseous hemangioma of the seventh cervical vertebra with osteoid formation mimicking metastasis: A case report. J Med Case Rep 2009;3(92):1–4.

[23] Wallis LA, Asch T, Maisel BW. Diffuse skeletal hemangiomatosis: report of two cases and review of literature. Am J Med 1964;37(4):545–63.

[24] Laguna R, Silva F, Vazquez-Selles J, Orduna E, Flores C. Vertebral hemangioma mimicking a metastatic bone lesion in well-differentiated thyroid carcinoma. Clin Nucl Med 2000;25(8):611–3.

[25] Kulshrestha M, Byrne P. Multiple primary haemangiomas of bone mimicking vertebral metastases. J R Soc Med 1997;90(11):632–4.

[26] Puri S, Gupta N, Asotra S. Hemangioma of rib masquerading a malignancy. J Cancer Res Ther 2018;14(10):809–11.

[27] Bellasri S, Fatihi J, Elktaibi A, El Asri A. Acute spinal cord compression caused by atypical vertebral hemangioma. J Craniovertebr Junction Spine 2017;8(3):275.

[28] Wallis LA, Asch T, Maisel BW. Diffuse skeletal hemangiomatosis. Am J Med 1964;37:545–63.

[29] Scolyer RA, Zhuang L, Palmer AA, Thompson JF, McCarthy SW. Combined naevus: A benign lesion frequently misdiagnosed both clinically and pathologically as melanoma. Pathology 2004;36(5):419–27.

[30] Fox MW, Onofrio BM. The natural history and management of symptomatic and asymptomatic vertebral hemangiomas. J Neurosurg 1993;78(1):36–45.

[31] Huvos A. Bone tumors: Diagnosis, treatment and prognosis, 2nd ed. Philadelphia, PA: WB Saunders, 1987.

SECTION FOUR: RADIATION THERAPY

In: Clinical Oncology
Editors: Ariel Tenenbaum et al.
ISBN: 978-1-53617-933-0

Chapter 10

USE OF SINGLE FRACTION PALLIATIVE RADIOTHERAPY FOR GASTRIC BLEEDING: A CASE REPORT

Leah Drost, Vithusha Ganesh, Bo Angela Wan and Edward Chow*
Odette Cancer Centre, Sunnybrook Health Sciences Centre,
University of Toronto, Toronto, Ontario, Canada

ABSTRACT

Palliative radiotherapy in fractionated courses is commonly used to treat bleeding due to gastric cancer. However, patient characteristics such as poor performance status, as well as disease-related symptoms can render prolonged courses of palliative radiation unfeasible. We report the case of a 93-year old man with severe bleeding and pyloric obstruction from an advanced stage gastric cancer, who was treated with a single fraction radiotherapy due to a poor performance status and symptom profile. This

* Corresponding Author: Professor Edward Chow MBBS, MSc, PhD, FRCPC Department of Radiation Oncology, Odette Cancer Centre, Sunnybrook Health Sciences Centre, 2075 Bayview Avenue, Toronto ON, Canada. E-mail: Edward.Chow@sunnybrook.ca.

case highlights the challenges associated with providing adequate symptom control in palliative patients with symptomatic gastric cancer.

INTRODUCTION

Gastric cancer currently ranks 4th worldwide in cancers most commonly diagnosed and 2nd in cancer-related mortalities (1-3). This malignancy is often difficult to detect in early stages, which contributes to its high mortality rate as it is often caught in advanced stages.

Gastric cancer can cause significant local symptoms such as bleeding, pain and obstruction (4). Specifically, gastrointestinal (GI) bleeding due to gastric cancer significantly impedes patient quality of life and can be life-threatening if severe. Several modalities can be used to treat symptomatic gastric cancer, including palliative chemotherapy, surgical resection, endoscopic hemostasis, and trans-catheter embolotherapy. In addition to these options, radiation offers a noninvasive method of palliation in this patient population. Radiation to control GI bleeding has been shown to be effective in achieving hemostasis when other treatment modalities are not an option, namely in patients whose poor performance status does not warrant a more invasive approach such as surgery or aggressive chemotherapy (5-6).

This report presents a case of an elderly man with newly diagnosed advanced stage gastric cancer causing severe GI bleeding and pyloric obstruction resulting in gastric distension.

CASE STORY

In January of 2017, a 93-year-old man with declining hemoglobin (53g/L) due to gastric bleeding was referred to the Rapid Response Radiotherapy Program, as an inpatient from another hospital.

An endoscopy and subsequent biopsy conducted in December 2016 confirmed a primary gastric adenocarcinoma. There was no evidence of metastases. The patient presented with a Karnofsky Performance Status of 40.

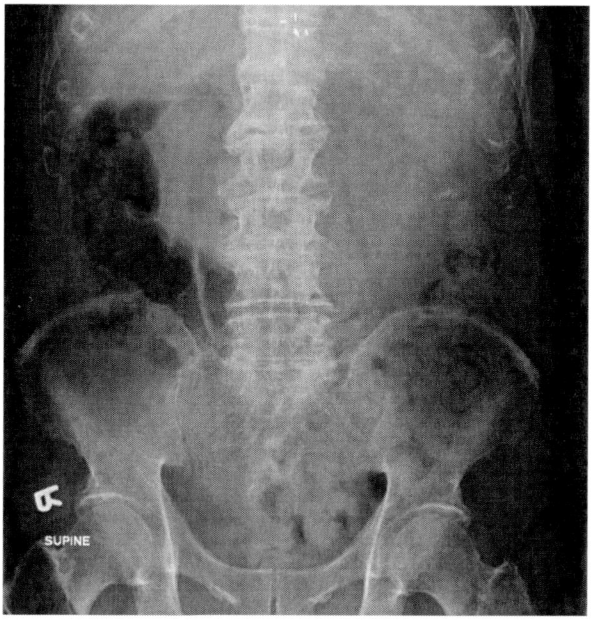

Figure 1. Gastrointestinal distension.

After careful consideration by the patient, his family, and several specialists, it was decided that palliative radiation was the best option for this patient, the intent of which was to control the severe GI bleeding. The patient was initially scheduled to receive 20 Gray in 5 fractions. However, when the patient arrived several days later for the first fraction of his treatment, it was noted that he was experiencing severe gastric distension (Figure 1) due to a pyloric obstruction from the primary tumor. It was decided that the patient would wait for several days and return to the radiotherapy once the distension had been relieved. After 3 days, however, the patient returned with distension that had progressed, and was experiencing significant pain and discomfort from this. Attempts to relieve the distention through maneuver of sitting positions and placement of nasogastric tube were unsuccessful. Due to the pressing matter of ongoing

GI bleeding progressively lowering the hemoglobin, the decision was made to re-plan the patient with a single dose of 8 Gray that day to the tumor causing pyloric obstruction with the aim of stopping the bleeding, relieving obstruction and lessening distension. The bleeding was halted with the radiation treatment and the patient eventually required bypass surgery for the pyloric obstruction. The patient unfortunately succumbed to the disease a few weeks later.

Discussion

Early gastric cancer is usually treated in an aggressive manner using approaches such as surgical resection, chemotherapy and/or radiation with a curative intent (6). Complications from this type of malignancy can include obstruction, bleeding, and pain (4, 6).

Our patient's case was complicated. Firstly, his GI bleeding was quite severe, as indicated by his low hemoglobin level. The patient also had several comorbid conditions and a poor performance status. In addition to the severe bleeding, this patient presented with extreme gastric distension caused by a pyloric obstruction (Figure 1). Pyloric obstruction is frequently mitigated with a surgical procedure such as a gastrectomy (7-8), however due to this patient's many complications an invasive procedure was decided against initially.

Before the gastric distension became clinically relevant, the patient was originally offered fractionated palliative radiotherapy to control the bleeding and relieve the obstruction. Radiation is indicated as an effective treatment option for bleeding and is often given as 30 Gray in 10 fractions in these cases; however, an optimal regimen has yet to be studied and established (5). While this prolonged course of radiation has been deemed adequate to control bleeding, it may not be a viable treatment option for palliative patients with poor performance status (9). In this patient's case, the initially prescribed radiation regimen became unfeasible for several reasons. His unstable and persistent gastric distention presented a challenge, and a more prolonged course of radiation would have required repeat imaging and planning of radiotherapy. This treatment plan would have placed high demands on the patient, and was not pursued given his poor performance status and frailty. Instead, to better accommodate the patient and the many complications presented in his case, single-fraction radiotherapy was offered and conducted.

Despite more evidence in support of prolonged courses of radiotherapy for GI bleeding, there is also evidence to indicate that short-course radiotherapy may be beneficial. In a retrospective analysis of 115 patients who received palliative radiation for symptomatic gastric cancer, Tey et al. reported a relatively high response rate of 81% for treatment of bleeding (4). They also noted no difference in response rates between low (≤39 Gy) and high (>39 Gy) dose regimens. Kawabata et al. conducted a retrospective review of 18 patients who received a total of 26 low-dose, short-courses (6 Gy in 3 fractions) to treat bleeding from unresectable gastric cancer (5). Based on their results, they suggested that a low-dose, short-course radiation was an effective and safe treatment option for this patient population.

CONCLUSION

This patient's case had many unanticipated complications, which made it difficult to offer treatment that would be traditionally given under better circumstances. However, this case also brings to light the need for more research on methods that mitigate unnecessary harm to patients who are difficult to treat. Specifically, more research on the efficacy of simpler, short-course radiotherapy for the treatment of GI bleeding should be conducted to confirm the use of this easier method.

ACKNOWLEDGMENTS

We thank the generous support of Bratty Family Fund, Michael and Karyn Goldstein Cancer Research Fund, Joey and Mary Furfari Cancer Research Fund, Pulenzas Cancer Research Fund, Joseph and Silvana Melara Cancer Research Fund, and Ofelia Cancer Research Fund.

REFERENCES

[1] Hu B, Hajj NE, Sittler S, Lammert N, Barnes R, Meloni-Ehrig A. Gastric cancer: Classification, histology and application of molecular pathology. J Gastroinest Oncol 2012;3(3):251-61.

[2] Patel TN, Roy S, Ravi R. Gastric cancer and related epigenetic alterations. Ecancer Med Sci 2017;11:714.

[3] Lu J, Cao L, Zheng C, Li P, Xie J, Wang J, et al. The preoperative frailty versus inflammation-based prognostic score: Which is better as an objective predictor for gastric cancer patients 80 years and older? Ann Surg Oncol 2017;24:754-62.

[4] Tey J, Choo BA, Leong CN, Loy EY, Wong LC, Lim K, et al. Clinical outcome of palliative radiotherapy for locally advanced symptomatic gastric cancer in the modern era. Medicine (Baltimore) 2014;93(22):e118.

[5] Kawabata H, Uno K, Yasuda K, Yamashita M. Experience of low-dose, short-course palliative radiotherapy for bleeding from unresectable gastric cancer. J Palliat Med 2017;20(2):177-80.

[6] Kondoh C, Shitara K, Nomura M, Takahari D, Ura T, Tachibana H, et al. Efficacy of palliative radiotherapy for gastric bleeding in patients with unresectable advanced gastric cancer: a retrospective cohort study. BMC Palliat Care 2015;14:37.

[7] Hussain T, Elahi B, McManus P, Mahapatra T, Kneeshaw PJ. Gastric obstruction secondary to metastatic breast cancer: a case report and literature review. J Med Case Rep 2012;6:232.

[8] Keranen I, Kylanpaa L, Udd M, Louhimo J, Lepisto A, Halttunen J et al. Gastric outlet obstruction in gastric cancer: a comparison of three palliative methods. J Surg Oncol 2013;108(8):537-41.

[9] Asakura H, Hashimoto T, Harada H, Mizumoto M, Furutani K, Hasuike N, et al. Palliative radiotherapy for bleeding from advanced gastric cancer: is a schedule of 30 Gy in 10 fractions adequate? J Cancer Res Clin Oncol 2011;137:125-30.

In: Clinical Oncology
Editors: Ariel Tenenbaum et al.
ISBN: 978-1-53617-933-0

Chapter 11

IS PRE-EXISTING NAUSEA AND VOMITING A BARRIER TO THE PROPHYLAXIS OF RADIATION-INDUCED NAUSEA AND VOMITING?

Shima Parsafar, Erin McKenzie, Dominic Chan, MBBS and Edward Chow*
Odette Cancer Centre, Sunnybrook Health Sciences Centre,
University of Toronto, Toronto, Canada

ABSTRACT

Radiation-induced nausea and vomiting (RINV) is commonly experienced by patients undergoing radiation to emetogenic regions and can negatively affect clinical outcomes and patient quality of life. There is little evidence surrounding optimal management of RINV in patients with pre-existing nausea and vomiting as these patients are often excluded from clinical trials. Recent studies have examined the efficacy

* Corresponding Author: MBBS. E-mail: Edward.Chow@sunnybrook.ca.

of managing RINV in this patient population with first generation 5-hydroxytryptamine receptor antagonists (5-HT3 RA) such as ondansetron, which demonstrated improvements in rates of overall control of nausea and vomiting. Additionally, the use of a second generation 5-HT3 RA, palonosetron, was investigated for management of RINV in patients with and without pre-existing nausea and vomiting. Results from two studies conducted at our center suggest palonosetron is safe and efficacious for RINV management as both patient groups experienced improved rates of complete control of nausea and vomiting. Further investigation, including phase III studies with larger sample sizes, are needed to expand our current knowledge base on the use of novel antiemetics for RINV such as palonosetron and best practices for the management of RINV in patients with pre-existing nausea and vomiting.

INTRODUCTION

Nausea and vomiting are commonly experienced by patients in advanced stages of cancer and can be a result of disease progression or adverse reactions related to cancer treatment. Radiation-induced nausea and vomiting (RINV) can occur as a result of radiotherapy to emetogenic regions and can cause significant distress to patients. A prospective observational trial by Maranzano et al. demonstrated that among 1020 patients undergoing radiation across 45 Italian radiation oncology centres, 11% (n=110) and 27% (n=272) of patients experienced vomiting and nausea, respectively (1). Other studies have estimated that nausea and vomiting may occur in up to 50-80% of patients when the upper abdomen is radiated (2, 3). Despite the high prevalence of this complication, several observational studies have shown that antiemetics were underutilized by clinicians and many were not aware of the availability of antiemetic guidelines (1, 4, 5). In one study, antiemetics were prescribed to only 17% of patients: 12.4% received prophylactic antiemetics while 4.6% received rescue therapy (1). RINV may lead to physical complications such as nutritional deficiency, weight loss, electrolyte imbalance and dehydration and has the potential to compromise clinical efficacy and overall survival through treatment delay, termination, or decreased compliance with concurrent therapies (6, 7). Additionally, a previous study by our group investigated the effect of RINV on quality of life (QoL) with the Functional Living Index-Emesis and found that during radiation, patients experiencing nausea had significant personal hardship ($p=0.003$) and trouble enjoying meals ($p<0.0001$) and those experiencing vomiting had decreased enjoyment of meals ($p<0.0001$) and imposed hardship on loved ones ($p=0.0004$) (8). In patients with pre-existing emesis, the negative effects of RINV on QoL may be magnified as the severity of their nausea and vomiting can increase during radiation.

It is suggested that the mechanism of RINV is similar to chemotherapy-induced nausea and vomiting (CINV) as both are thought to be related to damage of enterochromaffin cells in the gastrointestinal mucosa, caused by chemotherapeutic toxins or radiation (9). These cells release serotonin, activating 5-hydroxytryptamine 3 (5-HT3) receptors, which then send signals to the brainstem to produce an emetic response (9). The efficacy and safety of first generation 5-HT3 receptor antagonists (RA), such as ondansetron and granisetron, has been well-established in the management of CINV and RINV for the prophylaxis of nausea and vomiting. Moreover, results from an international survey of radiation oncologists indicated that first generation 5-HT3 RAs are the most common antiemetic agents prescribed by clinicians for prophylactic RINV management (10).

To determine the appropriate management of RINV, the American Society of Clinical Oncology (ASCO), Multinational Association of Supportive Care in Cancer/ European Society for Medical Oncology (MASCC/ESMO), and the National Comprehensive Cancer Network (NCCN) have developed antiemetic guidelines for radiotherapy regimens based on the emetic risk of the treatment areas. Table 1 displays the classification of emetic risk according to radiated site. The guidelines suggest the use of first generation 5-HT3 RAs such as ondansetron or granisetron for RINV prophylaxis for high and moderate risk regimens with or without the addition of dexamethasone (11–13). There is limited high level evidence investigating the proper management of low and minimal risk radiotherapy regimens and as such, recommendations for RINV management in these categories are less specific. The guidelines recommend the use of a first generation 5-HT3 RA, dexamethasone or a dopamine receptor antagonist for rescue treatment once an emetic event has occurred (11–13). The guidelines do not address management strategies for patients with pre-existing emesis as there is a lack of studies investigating this patient population. These patients are often excluded from antiemetic trials due to the belief that antiemetic agents are not as effective for this cohort.

Table 1. Emetogenic risk classification for RINV regimens

Risk Level	Risk of Emetic Event (%)	Site of radiation
High	> 90	Total body irradiation
Moderate	30-90	Upper abdomen, craniospinal
Low	10-30	Cranium, head and neck, thorax, pelvis
Minimal	< 10	Extremities, breast

CURRENT EVIDENCE

A previous study by Wong et al. investigating the use of an ondansetron rapidly dissolving film included a small sample of patients with pre-existing nausea and vomiting in a secondary prophylaxis group (n=4) (14). Rates of overall control for nausea and vomiting during the acute phase (days of radiation delivery to one day after radiotherapy completion) in the secondary prophylaxis group were both 100% and during the delayed phase (2-10 days after radiotherapy completion), they were 50% (14). This study demonstrated that patients with pre-existing nausea and vomiting before radiation benefited from a secondary prophylactic approach with the 5-HT3 RA, ondansetron.

A second generation 5-HT3 RA, palonosetron, has been approved for use in the management of CINV and is characterized by a higher selective binding affinity and a longer half-life, compared to ondansetron and granisetron (15). In a systematic review and meta-analysis of palonosetron use for CINV, palonosetron demonstrated superiority to other 5-HT3 RAs in the percentage of patients achieving a complete response (CR), complete control (CC), lack of emesis and lack of nausea (15). CR was defined as no emetic episodes and no use of rescue medications and CC was defined similarly, with the addition of no more than mild reported nausea. Due to its unique pharmacology, palonosetron is the only 5-HT3 RA at present to have a specific indication for the prevention of delayed CINV, attributable to the drug's longer half-life, which results in better control of nausea and vomiting after treatment completion. However, the utility of palonosetron in the prophylaxis of RINV is not well-established as few studies have been conducted in this area.

Our group previously conducted two pilot studies in order to evaluate the safety and efficacy of palonosetron for the management of RINV in patients undergoing palliative radiotherapy to sites with low and moderate emetic risk (16, 17). Patients received a single fractionation dose schedule of 8 Gy in 1 fraction or a multiple fractionation schedule of 20 Gy in 5 fractions or 30 Gy in 10 fractions and these groups were reported separately due to the increased potential for RINV with larger doses in the multiple fractionation schedules (16, 17). Patients were prescribed 0.5 mg oral palonosetron as prophylaxis at least one hour before the start of radiation treatment, and every other day until treatment completion with follow-up in acute and delayed phases (16, 17). The first study investigated palonosetron for the primary prophylaxis of RINV in patients without existing nausea and vomiting and the second study examined the efficacy of palonosetron for patients with pre-existing nausea or vomiting (16, 17).

For the study population consisting of patients without pre-existing nausea and vomiting, the primary endpoint was control of vomiting and secondary endpoints included control of nausea and QoL (16). In the acute phase, 93.3% and 74.7% of evaluable patients (n=75) reported CC of vomiting and nausea, respectively (16). In the delayed phase, 93.2% and 74.0% reported CC of vomiting and nausea, respectively (16). 2.7% of patients reported use of rescue medication due to a lack of CC (16). 95.5% of patients receiving a single fraction of radiation reported CC of vomiting and 84.1% reported CC of nausea in the acute phase (16). In the delayed phase, rates of CC of vomiting and nausea decreased to 90.7% and 69.7%, respectively (16). In the acute phase, patients who received multiple fractions of radiation, 90.3% and 61.3% reported CC of vomiting and nausea, respectively (16). In the delayed phase, rates of CC of vomiting and nausea increased to 96.7% and 80.0%, respectively (16). This study reported improved primary prophylaxis of RINV with palonosetron and noted few adverse events, suggesting it may be a safe and efficacious treatment for RINV.

The second study employed an identical study design, except enrollment of patients with pre-existing emesis was permitted. Prophylaxis and rescue (PR) was defined as a decrease in anti-emetic use, or episodes of nausea and/or vomiting from baseline (17). Complete prophylaxis (CP) was defined as no increase in anti-emetic use, or episodes of nausea and/or vomiting (17). Partial control (PC) was defined as an increase of 1–2 episodes of nausea or vomiting, or an increase in use of anti-emetic medication from baseline and an uncontrolled response was indicated by 3 or more episodes of nausea or vomiting (17). For enrolled patients (n=14) in the acute phase, 6 patients (42.9%) reported PR of nausea, 6 patients (42.9%) reported CP and 2 patients (14.3%) reported PC of nausea (17). Similarly, 3 (21.4%) and 10 patients (71.4%) experienced PR and CP of vomiting in the acute phase, respectively (17). One patient (7.1%) reported PC of vomiting in the acute phase (17). In the delayed phase (n=13), 6 patients (42.9%) reported PR, 1 patient (7.7%) reported CP of nausea and 1 patient (7.7%) reported PC of nausea (17). Four patients (30.8%) experienced an uncontrolled response, and 1 patient had incomplete data (17). Similarly, 2 patients (15.4%) reported PR, and 7 patients (53.8%) reported CP of vomiting (17). Two patients (15.4%) experienced PC, 1 patient (7.7%) reported an uncontrolled response, and 1 patient had incomplete data (17). This study concluded that palonosetron appears to be safe and efficacious for the secondary prophylaxis of RINV in patients with pre-existing nausea and vomiting.

Conclusion

Although patients with pre-existing nausea and vomiting have previously been excluded from clinical trials due to the perception of increased difficulty in symptom control, results from studies conducted at our center suggest that the use of 5-HT3 RAs such as ondansetron or palonosetron are safe and efficacious for the management of RINV in this population. In particular, palonosetron seems to demonstrate a superior potential to prevent RINV in patients with or without pre-existing emesis as well as promising improvement of symptoms and few adverse effects, ultimately, leading to improved patient QoL.

Further investigation through phase III studies with larger sample sizes are needed to advance our current knowledge surrounding the potential benefits of using palonosetron for RINV. With a greater body of evidence, effective management of patients with pre-existing nausea and vomiting can be elucidated through the establishment of more tailored guidelines for this patient population as well as the inclusion of potentially superior antiemetic treatments such as palonosetron.

Acknowledgments

We thank the generous support of Bratty Family Fund, Michael and Karyn Goldstein Cancer Research Fund, Joey and Mary Furfari Cancer Research Fund, Pulenzas Cancer Research Fund, Joseph and Silvana Melara Cancer Research Fund, and Ofelia Cancer Research Fund.

References

[1] Maranzano E, De Angelis V, Pergolizzi S, Lupattelli M, Frata P, Spagnesi S, et al. A prospective observational trial on emesis in radiotherapy: Analysis of 1020 patients recruited in 45 Italian radiation oncology centres. Radiother Oncol 2009;94(1):36–41.

[2] Priestman TJ, Priestman SG. An initial evaluation of nabilone in the control of radiotherapy-induced nausea and vomiting. Clin Radiol 1984;35(4):265–6.

[3] Danjoux CE, Rider WD, Fitzpatrick PJ. The acute radiation syndrome: A memorial to William Michael Court-Brown. Clin Radiol 1979;30(5):581–4.

[4] Dennis K, Zhang L, Lutz S, van Baardwijk A, van der Linden Y, Holt T, et al. International patterns of practice in the management of radiation therapy-induced nausea and vomiting. Int J Radiat Oncol Biol Phys 2012;84(1):e49-60.

[5] Dennis K, Zhang L, Lutz S, van der Linden Y, van Baardwijk A, Holt T, et al. International radiation oncology trainee decision making in the management of radiotherapy-induced nausea and vomiting. Support Care Cancer 2013;21(7):2041–8.

[6] Henriksson R, Lomberg H, Israelsson G, Zackrisson B, Franzén L. The effect of ondansetron on radiation-induced emesis and diarrhoea. Acta Oncol 1992;31(7):767–9.

[7] Priestman TJ. Controlling the toxicity of palliative radiotherapy: The role of 5-HT3 antagonists. Can J Oncol 1996;6(1):17–22.

[8] Yee C, Drost L, Zhang L, Wan BA, Ganesh V, Tsao M, et al. Impact of radiation-induced nausea and vomiting on quality of life. Support Care Cancer 2018;26(11):3959–66.

[9] Feyer PC, Stewart AL, Titlbach OJ. Aetiology and prevention of emesis induced by radiotherapy. Support Care Cancer 1998;6(3):253–60.

[10] Dennis K, Zhang L, Lutz S, van Baardwijk A, van der Linden Y, Holt T, et al. International patterns of practice in the management of radiation therapy-induced nausea and vomiting. Int J Radiat Oncol 2012;84(1):e49–60.

[11] Roila F, Molassiotis A, Herrstedt J, Aapro M, Gralla RJ, Bruera E, et al. 2016 MASCC and ESMO guideline update for the prevention of chemotherapy- and radiotherapy-induced nausea and vomiting and of nausea and vomiting in advanced cancer patients. Ann Oncol 2016;27(5):119–33.

[12] Hesketh PJ, Kris MG, Basch E, Bohlke K, Barbour SY, Clark-Snow RA, et al. Antiemetics: American Society of Clinical Oncology clinical practice guideline update. J Clin Oncol 2017;35(28):3240–61.

[13] Ettinger DS, Berger MJ, Aston J, Barbour S, Bergsbaken J, Brandt D, et al. NCCN Guidelines Version 3.2018 Panel Members: Antiemesis. 2018.

[14] Wong E, Pulenzas N, Bedard G, DeAngelis C, Zhang L, Tsao M, et al. Ondansetron rapidly dissolving film for the prophylactic treatment of radiation-induced nausea and vomiting-a pilot study. Curr Oncol 2015;22(3):199–210.

[15] Popovic M, Warr DG, DeAngelis C, Tsao M, Chan KKW, Poon M, et al. Efficacy and safety of palonosetron for the prophylaxis of chemotherapy-induced nausea and vomiting (CINV): a systematic review and meta-analysis of randomized controlled trials. Support Care Cancer 2014;22(6):1685–97.

[16] Ganesh V, Drost L, DeAngelis C, Wan BA, Pasetka M, Chan S, et al. A pilot study with palonosetron in the prophylaxis of radiation-induced nausea and vomiting. Ann Palliat Med 2018;7(2):211–20.

[17] Ganesh V, Chan S, Zhang L, Drost L, DeAngelis C, Wan BA, et al. Management of radiation-induced nausea and vomiting with palonosetron in patients with pre-existing emesis: A pilot study. Ann Palliat Med 2018;7(4):385–92.

SECTION FIVE: PILOT PROGRAMS

In: Clinical Oncology
Editors: Ariel Tenenbaum et al.
ISBN: 978-1-53617-933-0

Chapter 12

PERSONAL DEVICE TELEMEDICINE IN A HIGHLY SPECIALIZED CANCER CARE DELIVERY MODEL: A PILOT STUDY TO ASSESS FEASIBILITY AND IDENTIFICATION OF FUTURE POTENTIAL

Ethan Law, Erin McKenzie, and Calvin Law*, MD

Odette Cancer Centre, Sunnybrook Health Sciences Centre, University of Toronto, Toronto, Ontario, Canada

ABSTRACT

A six-month pilot was implemented using novel telemedicine technology that allowed direct connection to patients' personal device for the delivery of care within the setting of a regionalized, highly specialized

---

* Corresponding Author: Professor Calvin Law MD, MSc, FRCSC Sunnybrook Health Sciences Centre, University of Toronto, Toronto, Ontario, Canada. E-mail: calvin.law@sunnybrook.ca.

practice in hepato-pancreatic biliary surgical oncology. Administrative data was reviewed to examine patient and visit characteristics to understand where potential populations could be best served by integrating personal device telemedicine into this practice. Secondly, an in-depth interview with the healthcare provider was used to determine themes that focused on the benefits and barriers of personal device telemedicine in this setting. 22% of clinical visits moved from in person to personal device telemedicine in the first six months of this pilot project. Patient distance from regional cancer centre were as close as 1.1 km but also as far as 1851 km. Interview analysis found novel themes including synergy rather than just replacement of in person clinical visits, better integration of family and caregivers into clinical decision making, and that personal device telemedicine may become an important method to address equity in a publicly funded healthcare system. Personal device telemedicine is a feasible technology for integration into highly subspecialized care and offers important and novel advantages for both patients and their healthcare providers. Future success will require technological investments that focuses on integrating this technology deeper into clinical workflows to remove existing barriers to implementation.

INTRODUCTION

Regionalized, specialized care for complex cancer care, particularly cancer surgery, was organized in the province of Ontario over the last 10 years. This bold, public health care policy established centres of excellence that would promote enhanced outcomes by building volumes, inter-disciplinary teams and specialized multi-disciplinary case conferences. Hepato-pancreatic biliary (HPB) surgical oncology was one such example. Major health outcomes including mortality rates decreased following the establishment of the centres of excellence establishing this strategy at the forefront of Cancer Care Ontario (CCO), the agency responsible for cancer services in Ontario (1-3).

Not unexpectedly, new challenges arose, including repeated medical imaging, clustering of medical imaging at centres of excellence, and patient accessibility issues. Digital imaging repositories appear to be a solution in development, though accessibility remains a challenge (4).

Patients farther from specialized centres faced barriers to care through repeated long-distance travel which was further exacerbated by differences in socioeconomic status in rural areas (5).

The establishment of the Ontario Telemedicine Network (OTN), with new technologies that go beyond traditional specialized room-based point to point communications, has explored potential new solutions (6). OTN now allows a secure platform that bridges patients and their healthcare providers through personal devices such as smartphones that allow for interactions from any provider location to any patient location at any time of day. In addition, the system allows for six lines to be connected simultaneously, allowing participation of distant family members anywhere with internet connection to participate simultaneously in a healthcare interaction.

The purpose of this manuscript is to review a six-month pilot of this advanced telemedicine development in the setting of a specialized HPB practice delivered at a centre of excellence. This review seeks to better understand the potential impact and future directions for telemedicine care delivery to address the challenges of delivering regionalized, specialized cancer care.

OUR STUDY

A pilot project involving the introduction of personal device video conferencing into a single HPB practice, functioning after business hours (6 pm-10 pm/18:00-22:00) was initiated in May 2018 to explore alternative clinical care delivery models. Support for the pilot was provided through administrative funding at 0.2 full time equivalent (FTE) for clerical staff.

Inclusion criteria followed the pilot design. Patients' inclusion criteria included fluency in spoken English or availability of a translator to English at home, availability of an internet connected device with a front facing camera and microphone at home, physically stable patients requiring care focused on discussing results or making clinical care decisions and agreement to participate in a telemedicine format clinical visit. Exclusion criteria included patients requiring wound care, patients requiring surgical drain care and physically unstable patients who required physical assessments.

An administrative review of this service was commenced in January 2019 to explore utilization patterns of the pilot. The dataset included anonymized patient characteristics including age at telemedicine appointment, cancer diagnosis, and distance from the cancer centre. Distance was measured using Google Maps from postal code of patient residence to postal code of the cancer centre, with the software set to "avoid tolls" and departure time at 09:00h Eastern Standard Time (EST) on a Monday. The first option in Google Maps was then used to retrieve distance (kilometres) to cancer centre and time of travel (minutes).

Secondly, an exploratory interview with the surgeon leading the pilot was undertaken to explore novel qualitative themes exploring barriers and future potential for telemedicine in this setting. The interview was structured by key topics and enhanced by probes designed to elicit further themes. The interview was designed as a 60-minute recorded interview with answers reviewed after to carefully delineate themes elicited from each topic.

FINDINGS

Data between May 1, 2018 until December 31, 2018 was reviewed. During this pilot, there were a total of 1,047 patient visits to this specialized HPB practice. Of those visits, 230 (22%) were conducted through telemedicine technology using personal devices.

General characteristics of the patients enrolled in the pilot study are outlined in Table 1. The patients had a very wide range in age from 34 years to 91 years. Diagnosis at telemedicine visit involved 61.3% patients who were deemed having a primary cancer only and 38.7% having metastatic cancer.

Visit characteristics are outlined in Table 2. The median number of visits per patient was two, with the time per visit set by electronic schedule at 30 minutes. There were no variations in visit length due to the electronic timing of the video connection. Patient distance from the regional cancer centre had a range of 1.1 km to 1,851 km, with the median distance being 46.7 km. The driving time per Google Maps calculation ranged from three minutes to 1,171 minutes, with a median driving time of 35 minutes.

Table 1. Patient characteristics

Patient characteristic	**Result**
Study population (n)	112
Study visits (n)	230
Male: female gender ratio	60:52
Age (years), median (range)	61 (34 – 91)
Cancer site per visit	
Primary cancer	141 (61.3%)
Gastric	13 (5.7%)
Gallbladder	1 (0.4%)
Bile duct	21 (9.1%)
Liver	24 (10.4%)
Pancreas	48 (20.9%)
Small bowel	27 (11.7%)
Adrenal	7 (3.0%)
Metastatic cancer	89 (38.7%)

Table 2. Telemedicine visit characteristics

Visit characteristics	**Result**
Study visits (n)	230
Number of visits per patient, median (range)	2 (1-13)
Time per visit	30 minutes
Distance from regional cancer centre, median (range)	46.7 km (1.1 – 1851 km)
Driving time to regional cancer centre, median (range)	35 minutes (3 – 1171 minutes)

Interview results and themes

A 60-minute in-depth interview was undertaken with the surgeon (CL) involved in this study. Topics and themes generated under each topic are listed in Table 3. Important themes included many patient benefits, and several barriers that will be presented in further detail below.

Table 3. Interview topics and themes identified

Interview topic	Themes generated
Ability to deliver clinical care	– Synergy with standard in-person clinical care – Enhanced family and caregiver participation – Patient benefits regardless of age, or distance from regional cancer centre
Care efficiency	– Much more efficient for patients – Lower throughput for clinicians
Technology	– Adjunct technology required for telemedicine to work effectively – Still a barrier for access for some
Future potential	– Critical for future delivery of healthcare – An important tool for equity

Ability to deliver clinical care: Synergy with standard in person clinical care

There were repeated references to how telemedicine synergized rather than replaced standard in-person clinical care. Telemedicine was used prior to and following in-person meetings. Before an in-person clinical visit, telemedicine was offered to some new patient consults travelling from a great distance, where the initial meeting was conducted by personal device telemedicine, allowing not only a clinical discussion but also allowing some set-up of additional necessary investigations locally before the next clinical visit. It also allowed the consult to occur more rapidly as it was conducted outside of a typically filled standard clinic. After an in-person clinical visit, telemedicine was also offered to provide additional counseling time, or to include other family members that were not able to attend the in-person visit. There were many references to how this helped enhance patient understanding and informed decision making in some complex cancer care decisions.

Ability to deliver clinical care: Enhanced family and caregiver participation

As introduced above, the personal device telemedicine allowed for up to six other participants from other remote points to join in the telemedicine visit. This allowed for many enhanced family discussions and increased access to patient family members living in different cities, different provinces and even different countries in one case. The environment enhanced the discussion and allowed family members to ask their questions directly to the surgeon, thereby sparing the patient the burden of explaining complicated medical issues to their family and caregivers.

Ability to deliver clinical care: Patient benefits regardless of age or distance from regional cancer centre

Although telemedicine was generally offered to benefit patients living far away from cancer centres, there were multiple references to patients benefiting even if they lived very close. This telemedicine pilot used evening times, and thus many patients were able to take the time to participate in their healthcare decisions outside of business hours, saving them travel through avoiding busy traffic and saved them taking any time off work. Additionally, many family members and caregivers benefited from this time that allowed them to participate in their loved one's care without taking additional time off work. These themes were also reflected in questions regarding care efficiency.

Care efficiency: Much more efficient for patients

As stated above, the personal device telemedicine appointment times could be scheduled outside of regular business hours as it did not require attendance by the standard inter-professional medical and clerical staff at the time of the appointment. This resulted in appointment times that avoided patients' or their families and caregivers taking time off work. Furthermore, the electronic system was booked at 30-minute intervals which set a clearer expectation for the patient about the time parameters of their appointment. In return, it also resulted in the virtual system coming on line for every telemedicine appointment on time, saving many hours of "waiting room" time that were occurring at in-person visits.

Care efficiency: Much lower throughput for clinicians

Despite the improvements for patient efficiency, it was noted that for a given time period, there was less total volume of patient throughput for the clinician. This system prevented multiple clinic bookings at the same time slot, and occasionally the surgeon found that 30 minutes were in excess of what was required to discuss issues with the patient, and the time could not be then given to another patient, as would happen in a standard in person patient clinic.

Technology: Adjunct technology required for telemedicine to work effectively

Although personal device telemedicine technology was lauded, it was noted that it worked in the setting of a centre with access to documentation from a wide group of other centres and included an ability to access outside imaging. For personal device telemedicine to be translated to other practices and other jurisdictions, it was noted that there was a definite requirement for this level of technological connectivity to be in existence.

Technology: Still a barrier for access for some

It was repeated that some patients could not access this personal device telemedicine. There were still a large number of patients who did not have active email or access to high speed internet. Furthermore, there was a subset of patients who tested their system after agreeing initially to participate, but the testing protocol showed that their connection was not fast enough. Furthermore, during this pilot, an additional app had to be installed on their personal device in order to allow the system to work. It was noted that the system was going to be improved with no additional app necessary, and the ability to perform adequately using lower bandwidth but these changes were due to be launched after the study period.

Secondly, it was felt that the clinician involved at this time did need to be somewhat “technology savvy” and that another barrier would be the hesitation for clinicians to offer telemedicine due to their inability to adequately work with the current technology in place. Further work to “make the technology invisible” may solve this, but the current software has not yet achieved that state.

Future potential: Critical for future delivery of healthcare

Despite the barriers, there was a repeated theme that “this felt like the future of clinics.” It was acknowledged that the decrease in throughput could easily be addressed by moving many clinical appointments to physician extenders including nurse practitioners or physician assistants which could be done concurrently or independently from the surgeon-led clinic. However, the ability to separate predictable clinic visits that focused on important clinical conversations from the more unpredictable environment of the standard in-person clinic that included issues such as dressing changes was felt to be extremely beneficial for clinicians and patients alike.

Future potential: An important tool for equity

It was expressed in several instances that this tool allowed for many patients without the ability to easily attend in-person visits due to economic reasons such as travel or inability to take time off work, to participate in an in-depth clinical visit with a subspecialist. It allowed the subspecialist to offer additional counseling and discussion that would have previously been passed back to local general practitioners. This was felt to be an important tool for many populations that did not have equivalent access to care. It was referred to several times as "an important tool for equity" and that the full potential of this technology for this issue had not been fully explored.

Discussion

Telemedicine uses communication technology to provide healthcare to patients from a distance. This allows improved access to health care for those who can't make it to the hospital. These people include: rural area residents and patients that suffer physical limitations. Telemedicine originated with the creation of telecommunication technology, including the telegraph and the radio. It wasn't until the early 20th century that this technology was used for medical communication purposes. Dr Hugo Gernsback debuted with the first telemedicine device, called the "teledactyl." This tool was designed to allow the doctor to communicate to the patient from afar and provides the doctor a video feed of the patient. Even though the "teledactyl" never made it past the concept stage, it was the pioneer of telemedicine.

Today, telemedicine is advancing faster than it ever has before due to novel software platforms and devices. The rise of communication apps, such as Skype and Facetime, gave new ideas surrounding how to develop telemedicine with user-friendly interfaces and designs. In Ontario, a major issue in telemedicine was developing a system that would meet privacy regulations and thus an independent system was developed that not only facilitated a point to point type video streaming encounter, but would also be a scheduling system, and a platform for non-patient healthcare virtualization (7,8).

This early pilot study demonstrates some very novel advantages for telemedicine in a highly specialized cancer care delivery model. It helped demonstrate feasibility of a personal device system which further enhances patients' ability to access care when compared with older versions of telemedicine which still required patients to travel to a local "telemedicine studio." It also brought new emphasis to the fact that distance alone was not the only major advantage; the increased consistency of appointment times, facilitating family and caregiver participation, and synergy with standard in-person clinic visits either before or after are new, important factors that encourage the progressive integration of this technology into clinical care.

Finally, a very compelling theme was related to equity. In the process of improving outcomes in complex cancer care, regionalization of care was instituted and has demonstrated improved outcomes. However, regionalization predominantly fell to larger urban centres, pulling care farther away from populations outside of those regions, many of which were considered vulnerable populations with higher levels of isolation and lower socio-economic strata. Technology such as smartphones, featuring broadband access and ownership of personal devices with integrated video and audio allowed for an opportunity to address this lack of equity by removing barriers for patients in these vulnerable areas to provide better access to highly specialized care. This is a key factor in planning for the expansion of this technology, particularly in the setting of a publicly funded health care system built on the principle of allowing all inhabitants of its jurisdiction to have equal access to quality care (5).

Although this review examined a pilot study involving HPB surgery, the principles could be as readily applied to settings requiring any complex care such as drug addiction, chronic pain, or mental health. Furthermore, this system can act as an extender for specialized physicians. Combined with lower resource physician extenders at more locales, an entire healthcare system that better optimizes the limited subspecialized resources by extending their capacity may be ultimately more efficient than building more infrastructure or expanding human resources. These are important considerations for future healthcare sustainability.

Conclusion

This study helps explore a vast future that will be made possible through the implementation of personal device telemedicine. Our plan moving forward is to further explore this technology by including patient experience measures, cost utility studies and comparative studies to better understand the true impact on care delivery and efficiency, particularly in the setting of costly, highly specialized cancer care.

Acknowledgments

We thank the generous support of Bratty Family Fund, Michael and Karyn Goldstein Cancer Research Fund, Joey and Mary Furfari Cancer Research Fund, Pulenzas Cancer Research Fund, Joseph and Silvana Melara Cancer Research Fund, and Ofelia Cancer Research Fund.

References

[1] Marcaccio M, Langer B, Rumble B, Hunter A. Hepatic, pancreatic and biliary tract (HPB) surgical oncology standards. Cancer Care Ontario 2006 URL:

https://www.cancercareontario.ca/en/content/hepatic-pancreatic-and-biliary-tract-surgical-oncology-standards.

[2] Simunovic M, To T, Theriault M, Langer B. Relation between hospital surgical volume and outcome for pancreatic resection for neoplasm in a publicly funded health care system. CMAJ 1999;160(5):643-8.

[3] Kagedan DJ, Goyert N, Li Q, Paszat L, Kiss A, Earle CC, et al. The impact of increasing hospital volume on 90-Day postoperative outcomes following pancreaticoduodenectomy. J Gastrointest Surg 2017;21(3):506-15.

[4] Hallet J, Coburn NG, Alberga A, Fu L, Tharmalingam S, Beyfuss K, et al. Reducing repeat imaging in hepato-pancreatico-biliary surgical cancer care through shared diagnostic imaging repositories. HPB (Oxford) 2019;21(1):96-106.

[5] Hallet J, Law CH, Karanicolas PJ, Saskin R, Liu N, Singh S. Rural-urban disparities in incidence and outcomes of neuroendocrine tumors: A population-based analysis of 6271 cases. Cancer 2015;121(13):2214-21.

[6] EVisit. The ultimate telemedicine guide: What is telemedicine? EVisit 2018. URL: https://evisit.com/resources/what-is-telemedicine/.

[7] Greiwe M. Why your practice should never use Facetime or Skype for telemedicine. Ortholive 2018 URL: https://www.ortholive.com/blog/why-your-practice-should-never-use-facetime-or-skype-for-telemedicine.

[8] Milton C. Why not Skype, FaceTime, Google Hangouts video for telehealth. VSee 2013. URL: https://vsee.com/blog/dont-skype-google-video-chat-for-telehealth/.

In: Clinical Oncology
Editors: Ariel Tenenbaum et al.
ISBN: 978-1-53617-933-0

Chapter 13

THE PROTECTION MOTIVATION THEORY AND ITS IMPACT ON PROSTATE CANCER SCREENING IN GUYANA

Naomi N Modeste*[1,*]*, DrPH, Malcolm Cort*[2]*, PhD and Janice E McLean*[3]*, PhD

[1]School of Public Health, Loma Linda University, Loma Linda, California, United States of America
[2]Athens State University, Athens, Alabama, United States of America
[3]University of Phoenix, Phoenix, Arizona, United States of America

ABSTRACT

Prostate cancer is of grave concern to men and the wider community in Guyana, South America. Several studies among Black men have shown a greater risk of prostate cancer in this population, as seen by the incidence of the disease and early mortality. Although prostate cancer usually

* Corresponding Author: Naomi N Modeste, DrPH, Professor Emerita, School of Public Health, Loma Linda University, 24951 North Circle Drive, Nichol Hall 1511, Loma Linda, California 92350, United States. E-mail: nmodeste@llu.edu.

occurs in older men, younger Black men in their 40s and 50s are disproportionately affected as well. Objective: To identify factors related to early detection of prostate cancer among men ages 40-70 years old living in Guyana, through the use of a hybrid theoretical model. Secondly, to investigate why men might be or not be motivated to use the digital rectal examination (DRE) as a cancer screening modality for early detection and prevention of prostate cancer. Methods. A non-randomized descriptive population-based study of 254 males using a structured questionnaire. Results. The findings suggest that partner status was significantly ($p<.001$) related to societal norms, and were more likely to perceive prostate cancer as a serious threat, and had a positive attitude toward screening ($p<.001$). Men who experienced psychosocial barriers were less likely to have intentions to screen for prostate cancer. Conclusions: The hybrid model used in this study revealed potential barriers to screening for prostate cancer, the most effective being psycho-social in nature. Males in Guyana expressed embarrassment relative to the DRE, and would like to keep the experience a secret. Although some men perceived time as a barrier to screening, they were still inclined to screen within a year to detect cancer early. Health education programs can further help to improve male involvement in cancer screening.

INTRODUCTION

The investigation of the likelihood of engaging in health promoting behavior has long relied on the health belief model (HBM), which is often regarded as the "grandparent of all health behavior change models" (1). This model explains that people will likely carry out health-promoting behaviors if they feel susceptible to a certain health hazard; if they feel that the hazard is likely to be severe or serious; and if they feel that the benefits of their actions outweigh the costs (2, 3).

More recently such investigations have argued that models which have been developed from the HBM have a thematic concept in common; that is, they explain the motivation to protect oneself from disease by taking preventive action. Consequently, these models have collectively come to be known as the protection motivation theory, although this theory is dominated by fear as a motivating factor (4). Whereas, in the HBM, perceived susceptibility and perceived severity were seen as separate components, the protection motivation theory combines these two concepts into one, and presently characterize them as perceived threat (5). This family of models now known as protection motivation theory illustrates that factors involved in perceived threat combine to produce precautionary behavior, formerly called preventive health behaviors (1, 6).

A very prominent theory within the family of those which explain preventive health behavior is the Theory of Reasoned Action (TRA) (7). Since the data for the present study did not include a measure of perceived behavioral control, which is a part of the Theory of Planned Behavior (TPB), another model in the set of theoretical approaches which explain perceived threat (8), we draw from the TRA in building a model. This theory explains that intentions to perform preventive health behavior are a function of two factors; 1) the individual's attitude toward performing the preventive behavior, and 2) subjective/societal norms, which refer to the perceived social pressure from important others or institutions in which the individual may be embedded (7). In previous research, whether used within the TBA or TRA approaches, these two predictors have consistently shown strong predictive power across many health behaviors (9, 10). Specifically relevant to the present study, they have also shown usefulness in predicting cancer screening behavior among women (11), and among men, willingness to take a prostate specific antigen (PSA) test, and to take a DRE (5, 12)

The present research investigated reasons why males in Guyana may be motivated to utilize the digital rectal examination (DRE) as a screening modality for prostate cancer prevention. Research in this society on the use of this screening modality is absent from the literature. In an effort to avoid limiting the scope of this research we therefore utilized a hybrid model which includes parts of the HBM and the TRA (see Figure 1). We see this hybrid model as one that can be used to both identify the peculiarities of this societal context, and help to paint a profile of men who are likely to utilize the DRE as a screening modality for prostate cancer.

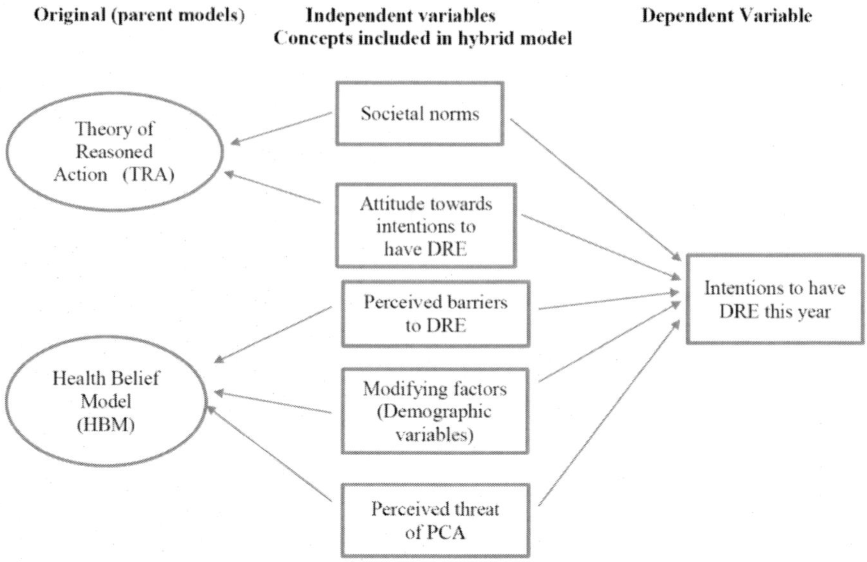

Figure 1. Hybrid model showing predictors of intentions to have DRE among Guyanese males.

OUR STUDY

This study was approved by the Loma Linda University Institutional Review Board (IRB). Data were collected with permission, from churches, and community health fairs in Guyana, using a structured questionnaire developed and pretested for this purpose. The population of interest was males 40 years and older, and every effort was made to target men of different demographics and counties. The original sample size was 273, but only 234 met the inclusion criteria after elimination of cases for missing data and being below the age criterion of 40 years. Only men who agreed to participate through oral consent, after reading or having the purpose of the study read and explained to them, were allowed in the study. Participants were informed not to write their names on the surveys. After completion of the surveys, they were placed in an envelope until time of data entry.

Analysis

Data were entered into a database, and analyzed using the Statistical Packages for the Social Sciences (SPSS) version 24. Descriptive statistics, bivariate correlations, and multivariate regression analyses were performed.

Variables

The dependent variable used in this study, intention to get screened, is the response to a statement "I intend to get a prostate exam this year." The response is a 5-point Likert scale coded from 1 = strongly disagree to 5 = strongly agree. The predictor variables used to operationalize the hybrid model can be identified by the original models from which they are derived (parent models). These variables are as follows:

- From the Health Belief Model – Two demographic variables were used as modifying factors, these are partner status and yearly household income. Partner status was coded to reflect partnered = 1; this category included males who were either married or living with a female partner. All others were grouped into a single category and coded as 0. Household income was grouped into six categories from $5k to over $50k per year. Perceived barriers to the DRE are as follows:
- Psycho-social barriers – this is a crude measure or additive scale which combined three questions about the DRE being embarrassing, being a violation of my masculinity, and keeping it a secret if I accept a DRE (used as a perception of stigma attached to this procedure). Cronbach's alpha reliability for this measure is .533. Single item variables used as perceived barriers include: time as a potential barrier – a response to the question about whether time is likely to prevent the respondent from getting a test to help

detect cancer early; fear of loss of sexual ability – a response to the question about whether surgery for prostate cancer can prevent a man from performing sexually; and perceived prostate cancer threat (PCA threat) – a response to the question about whether prostate cancer would be very serious if I get the disease. This variable is conceptualized as recognition of the threat that the disease poses to the health or life of the respondent. In this hybrid theory it is an aspect of the summary concept of perceived seriousness (along with perceived susceptibility – not used in this analysis) (5).

- From the theory of Reasoned Action (TRA) – From this parent model we used two constructs; societal norms and attitude towards the DRE. Societal norms refer to the perceived social pressure from important others or institutions in which individuals may be embedded. Attitude towards the behavior includes positive or negative feelings toward the behavior, which may spring from internal socialization about the behavior (7, 13). Societal norms are measured by a combination of two Likert-type variables: 1) Members of my immediate family think I should get a prostate cancer test, and 2) I will get tested for prostate cancer if my wife or girlfriend tells me to do so. The Cronbach's alpha for this measure is .67. Attitude towards the DRE is an additive measure consisting of six variables as follows: 1) I believe that a PSA test for prostate cancer can detect cancer early. 2) Early detection of prostate cancer may improve my chances of living longer. 3) I would screen for prostate cancer regularly if it were free. 4) I plan to get screened for prostate cancer in the future. 5) I believe prostate cancer screening is effective in finding cancer early and 6) I believe if found early, prostate cancer can be cured. Each variable was a Likert-type measure with 1 = strongly disagree to 5 = strongly agree. Cronbach's alpha is .70.

FINDINGS

In considering the findings of this study we first look to the by-variate analyses in Table 1. While this type of analysis is considered preliminary, in that it indicates which predictors can be treated as sufficiently important to be included in a multivariate (regression) analysis, it also offers an opportunity to examine the relationships between pairs of predictors, independent of their relationship to the dependent variable.

Table 1. Inter-correlations among variables in the hybrid model (N = 254)

	Variables	1	2	3	4	5	6	7	8	9
1	Partner status	----	-.087	-.021	.093	.051	.042	.186**	.242***	.089
2	Yearly income		------	.120	.134*	-.030	.045	.172**	.011	.090
3	Psycho-social barriers			------	-.085	.176**	.184**	-.103	.092	-.164***
4	Time as a barrier				------	-.025	.129*	.147*	.072	.193**
5	Loss of sexual ability					------	.088	-.043	.096	.163**
6	Perceived PCA threat						------	.227***	.413***	.285***
7	Attitude to screening							------	.517***	.481***
8	Societal norms								------	.405***
9	Intention to screen									------

Note:

* Correlations significant at the .05 level.

** Correlations significant at the .01 level.

*** Correlations significant at the .001 level.

Of importance firstly is the role of partner status. Partnered men are significantly more likely to have a positive attitude towards screening than those who are un-partnered. Partner status is also strongly related to societal norms, in that partnered men are more likely to abide by societal norms ($p < .001$). While this variable does not contribute much to other predictors it shows the importance of the presence of strong ties represented by wives or girlfriends, and members of the immediate families in the lives of men in this sample. Being influenced by the pressure of societal norms is strongly related to perceived prostate cancer threat, and also to attitude towards screening. Men who are influenced by societal norms are also more likely to perceive prostate cancer as a serious threat and to have a positive attitude towards screening ($p < .001$).

In terms of the relationship of most predictors to the dependent variable, intention to screen, men who perceive psycho-social barriers to screening such as being embarrassed, perceiving the test as a violation of their masculinity, or who are inclined to keep it a secret perhaps because of a perception of the act being stigmatized, are less likely to have intentions to screen. On the other hand, those who perceive time being a constraint, or who are afraid that if prostate cancer develops to the point of necessitating surgery they would not be able to perform sexually, are inclined to have intentions to screen in future. In addition, perceiving prostate cancer as a serious health threat, having a positive attitude towards the DRE, and being motivated by societal norms, all are associated with intentions to screen in future.

The effect of model variables on intentions to screen in the future

In model 1, the modifying factors (demographic variables) included in the model had only 2% of the variance in the dependent variable. However, they were included because of their association with attitude towards screening and societal norms in Table 1. However, when indicators from the HBM were added the variance explained increased by 14.8%, and when in model 3 the indicators from the TRA were included they explained 38.3% of variance, adding 21% more of the variance over model 2.

Table 2. Multiple linear regression models: Hybrid model predictors of intention to get a prostate screening this year (N = 254)

Predictors	Model 1	Model 2	Model 3
	β	β	β
HBM variables (Modifying factors)			
Partner status	.115	.072	-.037
Yearly Income	.123	.101	.055
HBM variables (Perceived barriers)			
Psycho-social barriers		-.197**	-.204***
Time as a barrier		.145*	.109*
Fear of loss of sexual ability		.086	.131*
Perceived PCA threat		.309***	.142*
TRA variables			
Attitude to screening			.377***
Societal norms			.196**
R^2	.026	.174[a]	.383[a]
Percentage R^2 change	------	.148[b]	.210[b]
N	234	234	234

Note: * $p < .05$, ** $p < .01$, *** $p < .001$.
[a] Significant R^2, [b] Significant increase in R^2.

The direct effects of the HBM showed that psycho-social barriers were related to intentions, in that men who experienced such barriers were less likely to have intentions to screen. Of some interest is the finding that men who thought that time was a barrier to screening still indicated that they would be willing to screen before the year was over (model 2). Another barrier that was not significant (analysis not shown) was economic barriers. It is rational to conceive that money would not be a barrier in this society because health care is universal or administered by the government and free to all citizens. Recognition of prostate cancer as a threat seemed to serve as a motivation for men in the sample to indicate that they would seek screening.

When the full model was considered (model 3), the TRA variables were shown to be very useful in predicting screening behavior among this sample. Psycho-social barriers increased in significance and fear of loss of sexual ability became slightly significant as a predictor of screening in the future. Perceived prostate cancer threat weakened as a predictor but still maintained some significance. The direct effects of the TRA model proved to be strong predictors. Attitude towards screening was the strongest predictor of intentions in the models. Societal norms also significantly predicted intentions to screen.

DISCUSSION

This study is descriptive in nature. Our main purpose was to identify psycho-social and structural characteristics in the lives of men who displayed intentions to utilize prostate cancer screening within the year of the interview. We utilized a hybrid model which contained variables from the HBM and the TRA. Our findings indicated that although some men considered time a barrier to screening behavior, they were still inclined to get screened that year. However, the most effective barriers to screening were psycho-social in nature. These consisted of being embarrassed by the procedure, perceiving the intervention as a violation of their masculinity, and being inclined to keep the procedure a secret after having received it. The inclination to keep the experience of the DRE a secret was not surprising. In many men's perspective this procedure may be associated with homosexuality, and homosexual behavior is considered extremely deviant in Guyana. There are still serious legal consequences for male homosexuality by law… discrimination and lack of social tolerance of gender and sexual identity minorities are premised upon cultural tradition, religious opposition and the law" (14). Consequently, association with any action that can be considered to fit into that class of behavior can be tainting and stigmatizing to those involved (15). This finding strongly suggests that the DRE is perhaps considered to fall into "bad company" in terms of its perception as being associated with homosexual expression.

Among variables of the HBM, the perceived threat of prostate cancer is also a strong motivator for prostate screening behavior. It seems that prostate cancer and prostate enlargement are perceived as related, in that enlargement is always caused by cancer. The combined measure utilizing these two variables (prostate cancer being very serious, and prostate enlargement being a common part of aging) is associated with an increased willingness to seek screening within the year. While the belief in causation is false, this confusion may be responsible for some amount of fear, which in turn may motivate screening behavior in this population.

By far, the strongest predictors of screening behavior are from the TRA variables. These two predictors alone contribute 21% of the explained variance in intention to screen. In previous studies, whether used within the TBA or TRA approaches, these two predictors have consistently shown strong predictive power across many health behaviors, and more specifically they have also shown usefulness in predicting cancer screening behavior among women and men (9, 10, 11, 18).

In achieving an appreciation for the strength of these TRA concepts it is important to appreciate the predictors by which they are operationalized. The operationalized concept attitude towards screening, includes predictors which point to a belief system of conviction about the efficacy of screening. For example it consists of among others, belief that a PSA test can detect cancer early; that early detection of prostate cancer may improve chances of living longer; and that if found early, the cancer can be cured. A common characteristic among these predictors is that they are amenable or open to improvement through well-structured health education programs. Societies in developing countries like Guyana stand to gain much in an effort to encourage men to become involved in prostate cancer screening with health education that encourages greater belief in this preventive intervention. We feel that targeted health education programs may go a far way towards changing attitudes if they can be implemented at sites where men gather in exclusive groups such as barber shops or other male-dominant gathering places.

The accompanying concept in this theoretical perspective is "societal (subjective) norms," which consists of two measures that capture the influence of important others in the lives of men. These influences are from immediate family or relatives, and female significant others, specifically wives or girlfriends. It is a widely accepted sociological concept that strong ties like family members are strongly influential in the health behavior decisions of many people. These ties can become large-scale patterns which have the power to change and direct the lives of groups of people in important ways. In his often-referenced seminal work on social network dynamics Granovetter (16) argues that "… small-scale interaction becomes translated into large-scale patterns, and these, in turn, feed back into small groups" (16). We are in agreement with this theoretical perspective that strong ties, represented by family members and wives and/or girlfriends can be a dynamic force with the power to encourage men to seek prostate cancer screening despite their psycho-social barriers of fear and embarrassment at the prospect of engaging in the procedure of screening with the DRE.

REFERENCES

[1] Fisher JD, Fisher WA. Theoretical approaches to individual-level change. In: Peterson J, DiClemente R, eds. Handbook of HIV prevention. New York: Springer, 2000:3-55.

[2] Becker MH. The health belief model and personal health behavior. Health Educ Monogr 1974;2:324-508.

[3] Rosenstock IM. Historical origins of the health belief model. Health Educ Behav 1974; 2(4):328-35.

[4] Norman P, Boer H, Seydel ER. Protection motivation theory. In: Norman P, Boer H, Seydel ER, eds. Predicting health behaviour: Research and practice with social cognition models. Buckingham: Open University Press, 2005:81-126.

[5] Luder H, Frede S, Kirby J, King K, Heaton P. Health beliefs describing patients enrolling in community pharmacy disease management programs. J Pharm Pract 2015;29(4):374-81.

[6] Gerrard M, Gibbons FX, Bushman BJ. Relation between perceived vulnerability to HIV and precautionary sexual behavior. Psychol Bull 1996;119(3):390-409.

[7] Fishbein M. A theory of reasoned action: Some applications and implications. Nebraska Symp Motivation 1980;27:65.

[8] Ajzen I. The theory of planned behavior. Organ Behav Hum Decision Pocesses 1991; 50(2):179-211.

[9] Conner M, Sparks P. Theory of planned behaviour and health behaviour. In: Conner M, Norman P, eds. Predicting health behavior. Research and practice with social cognition models, 2nd ed. Buckingham, England. Open University Press, 2005:171-222.

[10] Godin G, Kok G. The theory of planned behavior: a review of its applications to health-related behaviors. Am J Health Promot 1996;11(2):87-98.

[11] Cooke R, French DP. How well do the theory of reasoned action and theory of planned behaviour predict intentions and attendance at screening programmes? A meta-analysis. Psychol Health 2008;23(7):745-65.

[12] Berglund G, Nilsson S, Nordin K. Intention to test for prostate cancer. Eur J Cancer 2005;41(7):990-7.

[13] Cort MA, Ramirez O, Chama S. Predicting sexual abstinence among Seventh-day Adventist emerging adults. Soc Sci J 2016;53:199-208. doi.org/10.1016/j.soscij. 2016.02.010.

[14] Giles L. CADRES Survey is an important vacuum in LBGT examination. Kaieteur New, 2013 Jul 20.

[15] Misir P. HIV and AIDS: Knowledge and stigma in Guyana. Kingston: University of the West Indies Press, 2013.

[16] Granovetter MS. The strength of weak ties. Am J Sociol 1973;8(6):1360-80.

[17] Sieverding M, Matterne U, Ciccarello L. What role do social norms play in the context of men's cancer screening intention and behavior? Application of an extended theory of planned behavior. Health Psychol 2010;29(1):72.

[18] Soskolne V, Marie S, Manor O. Beliefs, recommendations and intentions are important explanatory factors of mammography screening behavior among Muslim Arab women in Israel. Health Educ Res 2007;22(5):665-76.

In: Clinical Oncology
Editors: Ariel Tenenbaum et al.
ISBN: 978-1-53617-933-0

Chapter 14

COST ANALYSIS OF METASTATIC NON-SMALL CELL LUNG CANCER (NSCLC) AFTER COMPLETION OF CHEMOTHERAPY WITH THE INTRODUCTION OF ERLOTINIB

Rashid Ahmed[1,2,*], PhD, Sri Navaratnam[3], PhD and Tooba Ahmed[2]

[1]College of Nursing and Professional Disciplines,
University of North Dakota, Grand Forks, North Dakota,
United States of America
[2]Department of Community Health Sciences,
University of Manitoba, Winnipeg, Canada
[3]Cancer Care Manitoba, Winnipeg, Canada

ABSTRACT

Erlotinib has been funded for use as a second and third line treatment of advanced NSCLC since 2006 in Manitoba, Canada. The present paper

[*] Corresponding Author's E-mail: rashid.ahmed@und.edu.

outlines the cost effectiveness of Erlotinib by examining population-based total costs, service utilization, and clinical outcomes of patients with metastatic NSCLC receiving Erlotinib were explored from the time they completed chemotherapy till the end of follow-up date (31Dec2012), death, or relocation. Metastatic NSCLC patients, who were approved for Erlotinib in Manitoba between June 2006 and 31 Dec 2012, were selected. The Manitoba Cancer Registry (MCR) and chart review were used to capture the information on treatment and clinical outcome. Service utilization information and direct cost information were extracted from the electronic health records known as ARIA, the Physicians Claims, the Hospital Discharge database, and the Drug Program Information Network. Survival rate, using the Kaplan-Meier method, was calculated from the date of the Erlotinib approval date till end of follow-up date, Dec 31, 2012, or death. The median survival rate was 40.1 weeks. The average cost per patient was CA$30,503 and CA$987 per patient-week for patients who received Erlotinib. Ninety percent of the cost was accounted for by hospital stays and drug costs. General demographic patterns per cost suggested that current smokers tended to incur higher costs compared to non-smokers. The results of this study appear to replicate patterns of other studies examining the cost effectiveness such that Erlotinib appears to have a high survival rate paired with lower costs related to side effect management.

INTRODUCTION

Worldwide, lung cancer is the most common cause of cancer death (17.8% of all deaths) (1). Its incidence rate has increased by 20% since 1990 (2). The majority (85%) of new cases were non-small cell lung cancer (NSCLC) (2, 3) and approximately 50-65% are advanced-stage (Stage IIIb/IV) at presentation (4). We recently examined the 20-year outcome of non-small cell lung cancer in an international cancer benchmark study in Manitoba. Results indicated an improvement in survival over the last decade (5), with a 5-year probability of survival of 19% (6). However, such rates need to be placed within the context of healthcare costs in order to fully understand how treatments can benefit patients. The present paper examines the cost of Erlotinib within the Manitoba health care system.

Advances in technology and of cancer biology have led to the introduction of a variety of new diagnostics and treatments in oncology.

Chemotherapy improves overall survival and quality of life in advanced NSCLC (7) and some agents, like docetaxel and pemetrexed, have shown a survival advantage as the second line therapy (8). However, such treatments are associated with side effects such as anemia and febrile neutropenia (25). Erlotinib, a more recently developed second line treatment of NSCLC, has started to address ways inhibit epidermal growth factor receptor (EGFR)-tyrosine kinase during second and third line therapy (9; European Medicines Agency). As a secondary benefit, use of Erlotinib has been linked with less intrusive side effects as compared to traditional second line treatments such as Doxetacel and Pemetrexed (25). The differences in side effects between Erlotinib and typical second line treatments likely influences both the quality of life for patients, and costs related to addressing side effects. This is especially relevant given the high cost of intervention. Less side effects means higher quality of life and less healthcare costs to manage intrusive side effects.

Traditionally, randomized clinical trials (RCT) have been accepted as the gold standard of evidence to evaluate clinical efficacy and cost. In light of growing drug costs, cost effectiveness analyses based on RCTs have become necessary before the drug can be introduced to the market. RCTs may not necessarily reflect the real-world practice due to the need for standardized patients, and tightly controlled experimental protocols. As a result, cost effectiveness as measured by RCTs may not reflect the performance of a drug among a group of actual heterogeneous patients. Accurate estimation of drug effectiveness and its cost effectiveness is best done by performing a population based study.

Population based studies addressing Erlotinib have started emerging to determine its cost effectiveness within the contexts of health care systems by utilizing real world variables such as Quality Adjusted Life Years (QALYs), probability of cost effectiveness, life gained, and total costs. Results suggest that Erlotinib is linked with higher QALYs (25, 26), 25-93% probability of cost effectiveness (25, 26), and lower costs related to management of side effects (Carlson). While one study found higher overall cost for Erlotinib, this relative increase in monetary cost was offset by QALYs (26). Cost benefit studies of Erlotinib estimated overall cost for

Erlotinib ranging from approximately CA$17,000 to CA$50,000, and 25-95% chance of cost effectiveness (25, 26). It is important to note that many of these studies derived results from different countries with different healthcare systems (UK, Germany, US, Spain, etc.), suggesting that it is essential to look at the costs and benefits of Erlotinib within provincial health care system. This paper expands upon the current literature by presenting cost analysis of the patients who have used Erlotinib in the Province of Manitoba from 2006 to until December 2012 after completion of chemotherapy using the unique administrative database in Manitoba.

OUR STUDY

The Province of Manitoba has a large number of databases that were used to obtain information for this study. This administrative database has been previously described (11, 12). Data obtained included physician visits, services by billing tariffs, and diagnostic codes (ICD). The electronic database of Manitoba's Drug Program Information Network (DPIN) records every prescription drug dispensed to all Manitoba residents since 1995. The Manitoba Cancer Registry (MCR) was established in 1956, and all the neoplastic diagnoses are collected through mandatory reporting. The MCR also captures demographic data, treatment and staging information, and the personal health identification number, which is available for all who are covered by the provincial health care plan. Correspondence between the database was achieved by utilizing personal health identification numbers.

Patients

Cancer Care Manitoba (CCMB) has funded Erlotinib for use as a second or third line treatment of advanced NSCLC since June 2006. Demographic information of patients who were approved for the use of Erlotinib in the

Province of Manitoba diagnosed with trachea, bronchus, and lung cancer (ICD-9 162) were filed in the department of Pharmacy at Cancer Care Manitoba. Patients who were approved therapy between June 2006 and December 2012 were selected for the analysis.

Study design and cost analysis

A retrospective medical record search was performed to measure total direct cost and service utilization. The sources included the Manitoba Cancer Registry, ARIA (electronic chart review), the Physician Claims database, the Hospital Discharge database, and the Drug Program Information Network (DPIN) database.

All available service and treatment information from the diagnosis date of the last chemotherapy to end of follow up was obtained through review of electronic patient charts. End of follow date was selected from the earliest data from December 31, 2012, death date, or date moved out of Manitoba. Patients were tracked from the first use of Erlotinib until end date, even for patients with more than one approval date. Majority of patients (n = 169) follow up periods ranged from 5 to 598 days. A smaller portion of patients (n = 8) had notably long follow up periods ranging from 638 days to 1,516 days. These charts were also used to determine intended treatment line and details on previous chemotherapy. Survival was calculated using the Kaplan-Meier method from the date of the Erlotinib approval date to either death or end of the study (December, 2012).

This study provides population-based estimates of the total cost of all health resources consumed by patients using their historical charts from the perspective of the Manitoba health care system, and expressed in 2014 Canadian dollars. These resources include the cost of chemotherapeutic drugs, radiation therapy, physician appointments, diagnostic tests, and hospitalization costs covered by the Manitoba Health Plan; and drugs covered under the provincial Pharma Care plan.

Table 1. Demographic characteristics organized by gender

	Female		Male		Total
	Count	Col %	Count	Col %	Count
Diagnosis Age					
<55	31	31.96%	22	27.50%	53
55-64	39	40.21%	32	40.00%	71
65+	27	27.84%	26	32.50%	53
Stage					
Stage III	32	32.99%	22	27.50%	54
Stage IV	65	67.01%	58	72.50%	123
Histology					
Adenocarcinomas	69	71.13%	44	55.00%	113
Squamous cell	7	7.22%	9	11.25%	16
Large cell	21	21.65%	27	33.75%	48
Smoking History					
unknown	28	28.87%	26	32.50%	54
Non-Smoker	15	15.46%	5	6.25%	20
ex-Smoker	25	25.77%	23	28.75%	48
Smoker	29	29.90%	26	32.50%	55
1st Line Chemo Agents					
other	6	6.19%	8	10.00%	14
Platin-Gem	46	47.42%	40	50.00%	86
Platin-Pax	16	16.49%	12	15.00%	28
Platin-Vin	18	18.56%	16	20.00%	34
none	11	11.34%	4	5.00%	15
Intended Treatment Line					
1	11	11.34%	4	5.00%	15
2	37	38.14%	27	33.75%	64
3	46	47.42%	44	55.00%	90
4	3	3.09%	5	6.25%	8
with Hospitalization					
0	15	15.46%	14	17.50%	29
1	82	84.54%	66	82.50%	148
with Hospital ER entry					
0	48	49.48%	39	48.75%	87
1	49	50.52%	41	51.25%	90
CCI Score Group					
CCI count = 1	29	29.90%	23	28.75%	52
CCI count = 2	48	49.48%	32	40.00%	80
CCI count = 3	18	18.56%	17	21.25%	35
CCI count > 3	2	2.06%	8	10.00%	10

Cost estimates for each patient were obtained by multiplying resource quantities by their corresponding unit costs. Hospitalization cost was measured by multiplying the Resource Intensity Weights (RIWs) by hospital-specific mean case costs in Manitoba in the year 2014, which was $5,374. Wide ranges of variables were examined in order to investigate associated costs with patient characteristics (see table 1). Variables included gender, age of diagnosis, stage of cancer, histology, smoking history, first line of chemotherapy treatment, hospitalization, and Charlson Comorbidity Index (CCI). Age of diagnosis included three age groups: under 55, 55 to 64, and 65 and over. Stage of cancer included patients diagnosed with both stage III and stage IV NSLC, and histology included adenocarcinomas, squamous cell and large cell. Smoking history was categorized as non-smoker, former smoker, smoker, and unknown. Individuals without a smoking history noted in the patient chart were categorized as other (n = 54, 30.51%). First line of treatment was derived by extracting the chemotherapy started within the first 9 months since diagnosis and lasting for six months. First line chemotherapy agents included Platin-Gem, Platin-Pax, Platin-Vin, other, and none. Approval dates for Erlotinib were calculated in order to determine the treatment line, all cases categorized as second line treatment were administered at least 30 days after first line chemotherapy. Hospitalization was coded for both emergency room visits and hospital admittance. CCI was calculated utilizing conditions present 1 year prior to Erlotinib by using hospital discharge data and medical claims data.

Since the study was retrospective, future costs were not calculated and discounting was therefore not appropriate. A sample size calculation was not performed since the entire population eligible within the described timeframe was included. The analysis were carried out by SAS 9.4 statistical software package. The protocol was approved by the ethics review board at the University of Manitoba and Cancer Care Manitoba.

FINDINGS

There were 260 patients approved for Erlotinib in Manitoba between June 2006 and December 2012. Among the sample, 201 patients were diagnosed with stage III/IV lung cancer. A small proportion of the sample (n = 22) did not fill their prescription or lacked a recorded Erlotinib drug claim in the DPIN data until 2012. Two patients with different histology codes (80003 and 80013) were excluded from analysis. After eliminating patients that did not fit the intended criteria, 177 patients remained (see table 1 for demographic characteristics). The final sample included slightly more females (54.80%, n = 97) than males (45.02%, n = 80), with approximately 70% of the sample falling in the 55 and older range. Most of the sample was in stage IV of cancer (approximately 70%), and had adenocarcinomas histology (approximately 63%). In terms of smoking status, 31.07% (n = 55) smoked, 27.12% (n = 48) quit smoking, 11.30% (n = 20) never smoked, and 30.51% (n = 54) had an unknown smoking status. Majority of the sample received Erlotinib as a third line of treatment (50.85%, n = 90). A smaller portion received Erlotinib as a first (8.47%, n = 15), second (36.16%, n = 64), and fourth line treatment (4.52%, n = 8). First line treatments included receiving Platin-Gem (48.59%, n = 86), Platin-Vin (19.21%, n = 34), and Platin-Pax (15.82%, n = 28). Two patients were given the agent as the first line treatment after obtaining special approval from the pharmacy and therapeutics committee at Cancer Care Manitoba. Treating physicians' assessment was that these patients would not tolerate chemotherapy and recommended Erlotinib since their clinical profile suggested a favorable response to Erlotinib. Many participants were prescribed Erlotinib while admitted to the hospital (83.62%, n = 148), and approximately 50% of the sample was admitted to the hospital during treatment through a visit to the emergency room (n = 90). Majority of the sample had at least two comorbid issues at initial presentation (45.20%, n = 80) and smaller portion of the sample experienced one comorbid issue (29.38%, n = 52), three comorbid issues (19.77%, n = 35), and more than three comorbid issues (5.65%, n = 10).

Clinical outcomes

Clinical outcomes were examined with a smaller portion of the sample (N = 71). The median survival of this cohort was 40.1 weeks from approval date of Erlotinib. The mean survival was 54.8 weeks (40.8 for males; 62.6 for females). One-year survival was 25.4%; two-year survival was 5.7%. In our previous study (12), prior to the introduction of Erlotinib, the median (mean) survival was 17.8 weeks (30.0 weeks) from time of last chemotherapy with one- and two-year survival of 18.9 and 5.3 respectively. Introduction of Erlotinib increased the median (mean) survival by 22.3 weeks (24.8 weeks) compared to no further cancer treatment after the completion of chemotherapy. It has to be cautioned that this is a historical comparison of the median survival. To address possible bias in the estimated survival rate, we conducted the survival analysis excluding the two patients who had Erlotinib as a first line treatment. The remaining sample received Erlotinib as second or third line treatment. There was little change; without these two patients, median survival was 41.6 weeks from the Erlotinib approval (40.1 for males and 52.1 for females).

In order to examine the extent to Erlotinib related to higher survival by demographic variables, a cox proportion hazard model was conducted (see Table 2). There were no significant differences seen between collaborative stage, age group, patients with hospital ER entry, a specific histology, or smoking history. There was a significantly higher survival among those treated with Plantin-Gem (adjusted hazard ratio (AHR) = 1.82). There was a significant difference between survival rates of men and women, such that women treated with Erlotinib tended to have higher survival rales (AOR = 1.54: male compared to female).

Table 2. Stage III/IV lung cancer after Erlotinib approval overall survival model

	Crude Hazard Ratio	95% CI	P Value	Adjusted Hazard Ratio	95% CI	P-Value
Collaborative Stage			0.56			0.55
Stage III	1	Ref		1	Ref	
Stage IV	1.11	0.8- 1.6		1 .1	0.8 - 1.7	
Age Group			0.38			0.45
< 55	1	Ref		1	Ref	
55-64	1.12	0.8 - 1.7		1.07	0.7 - 1.6	
65+	0.85	0.6 - 1.3		0.82	0.5 - 1.3	
1st Line Chemo Agents			0.01			0.01
Platin-Gem	1	Ref		1	Ref	
Platin-Pax	1.09	0.7 - 1.7		1.12	0.7 - 1.8	
Platin-Vin	1.99	1.3 - 3.1		1.83	1.1 - 3.0	
none	2.13	1.2 - 3.8		2.41	1.3 - 4.5	
other	1.37	0.8 - 2.5		1.40	0.7 - 2.9	
Gender			0.01			0.02
Female	1	Ref		1	Ref	
Male	1.53	1.1 - 2.1		1.54	1.1 - 2.2	
With Hospital ER Entry			0.02			0.12
No	1	Ref		1	Ref	
Yes	1.47	1.0 - 2.0		1.32	0.9 - 1.9	
Histology			0.33			0.74
Adenocarcinomas	1	Ref		1	Ref	
Large cell	1.08	0.8 - 1.6		0.99	0.7 - 1.5	
Squamous cell	1.52	0.9 - 2.6		1.24	0.7 - 2.2	
Smoking History			0.13			0.35
Non-Smoker	1	Ref		1	Ref	
Smoker	1.87	1.0 - 3.4		1.56	0.8 - 2.9	
ex-Smoker	1.76	1.0 - 3.2		1.40	0.7 - 2.7	
unknown	2.02	1.1 - 3.6		1.75	0.9 - 3.3	

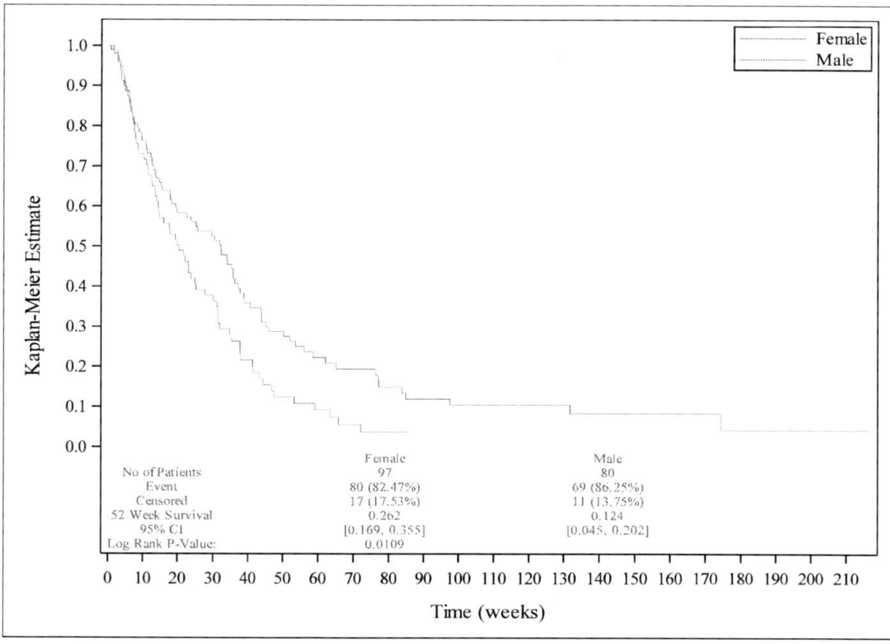

Figure 1. Stage III/IV lung cancer after Erlotinib approval overall survival Kaplan-Meier survival estimate by gender.

Kaplan-Meier estimates were utilized to estimate survival durations for patients on Erlotinib across variables such as gender, age group, stage of cancer, histology, smoking status, and first line of treatment (see Figures 1-6). Kaplan-Meier curves suggested that females had a higher probability of surviving for a longer period compared to males (see Figure 1). Those 55-64 had the highest probability of surviving compared to those 55 and younger, and those 65 and over (see Figure 2). Those with Stage IV cancer tended to have a longer probability of survival compared to those with stage three cancer (Figure 3). Individuals with the Squamous cell histology tended to have a higher probability of survival over time compared to those with large cell histology or Adeb carcinomas histology (Figure 4). Nonsmokers had the longest probability of survival compared to those with actively smoking, former smokers, or those with an unknown smoking status (Figure 5). Finally, Individuals receiving Platin-Gem as their first line of treatment compared to Platin-Pax, Platin-Vin (Figure 6).

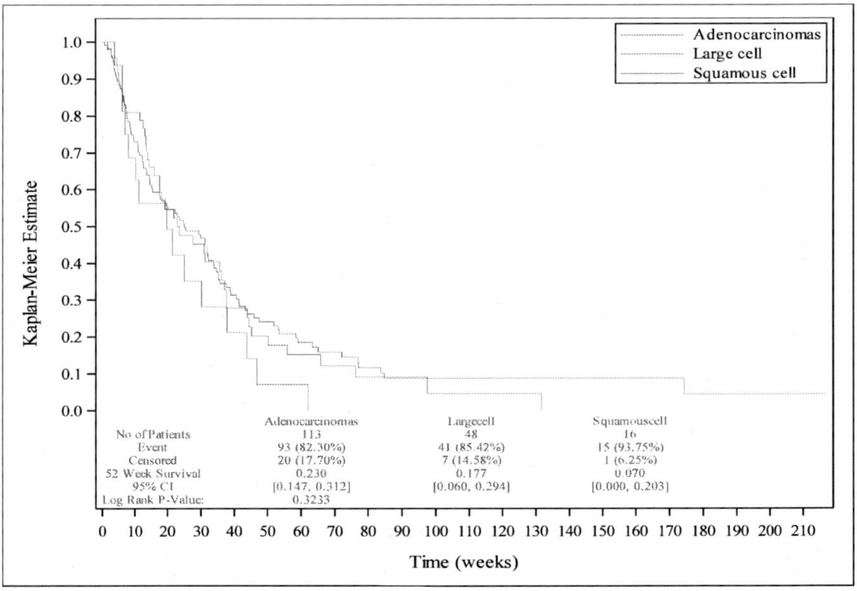

Figure 2. Stage III/IV lung cancer after Erlotinib approval overall survival Kaplan-Meier survival estimate by age group.

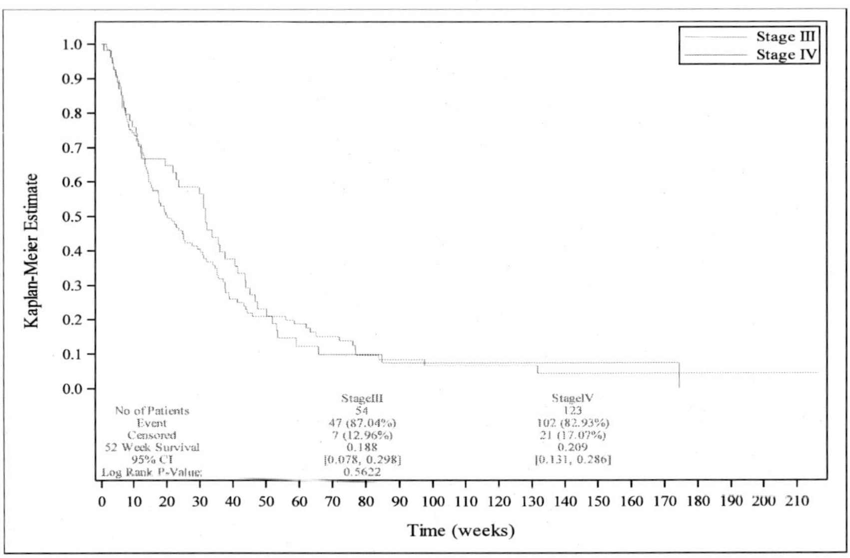

Figure 3. Stage III/IV lung cancer after Erlotinib approval overall survival Kaplan-Meier survival estimate by stage.

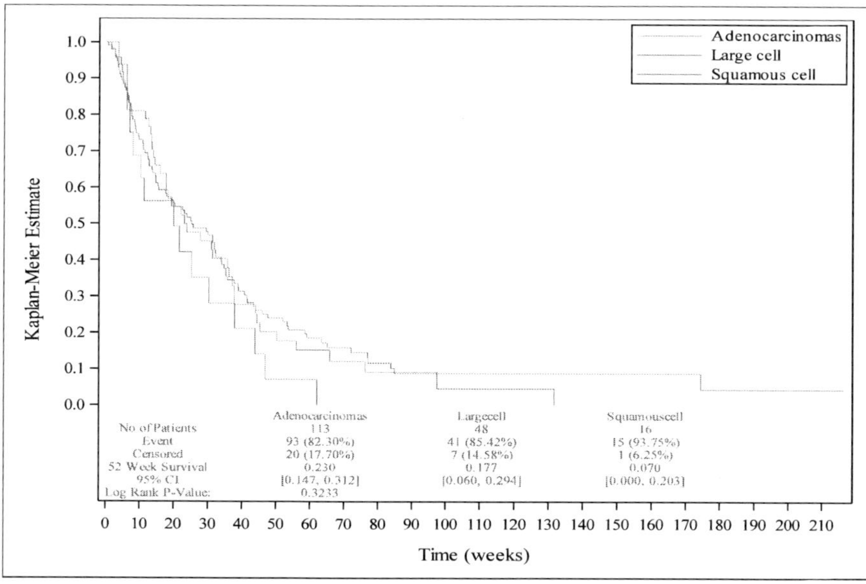

Figure 4. Stage III/IV lung cancer after Erlotinib approval overall survival Kaplan-Meier survival estimate by histology.

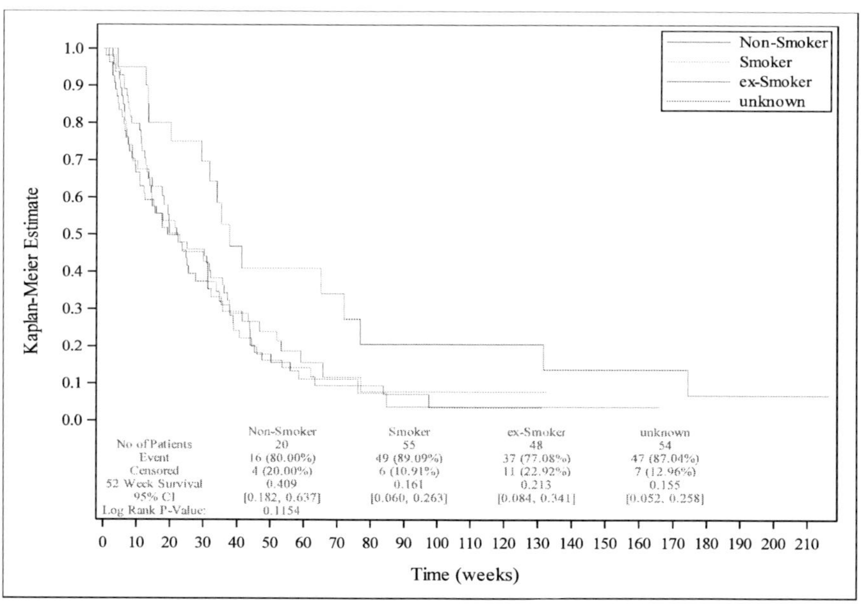

Figure 5. Stage III/IV lung cancer after Erlotinib approval overall survival Kaplan-Meier survival estimate by smoking status.

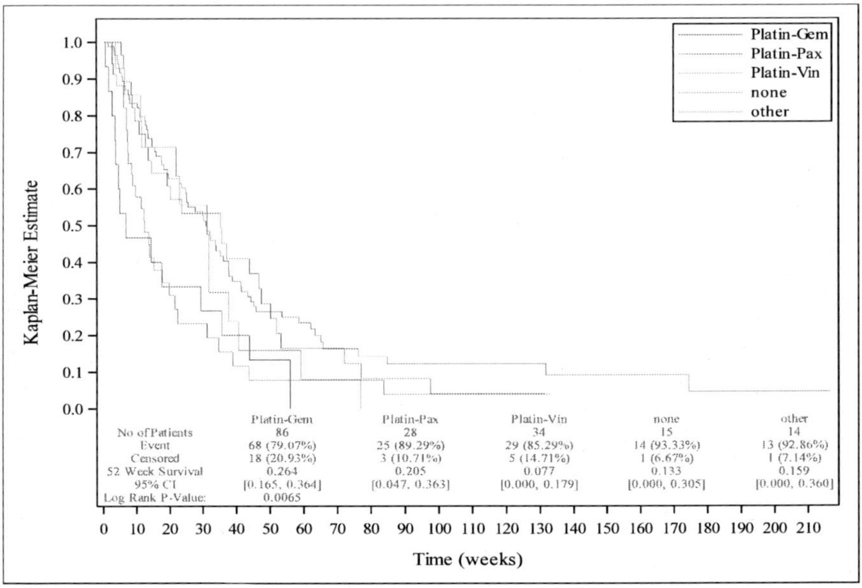

Figure 6. Stage III/IV lung cancer after Erlotinib approval overall survival Kaplan-Meier survival estimate by first line treatment.

Services utilization

The average number of medical claims was 26.5 claims per person (20.3 for males; 31.6 for females) or approximately 0.9 medical claims per person week. The average number of hospitalizations was 1.5 per person or about 0.05 cases per person week (5 cases per 100 person weeks). The average number of prescriptions filled was 43.8 per person (34.2 for males; 51.7 for females) or about 1.4 prescriptions per person week. Based on distributions, it appears that patients in the group less than 55 years of age are utilizing more services than the older population.

Costs

This is also evident in the average cost per patient-month disaggregated by cost resources. Calculated from the completion of the last chemotherapy cycle, the average cost per patient was $30,991 and average cost per patient-week was $2,582 as shown in Table 3.

Table 3. Total cost measured since approval date of Erlotinib by demographic characteristics

	Mean Cost (95% CI)	Median Cost (95% CI)	90th Cost (95% CI)
Total	$30,991 ($26,598-$35,384)	$22,029 ($18,762-$25,735)	$68,661 ($48,642-$88,170)
Gender			
Female	$34,122 ($27,536-$40,708)	$24,108 ($18,762-$30,635)	$80,873 ($55,776-$97,446)
Male	$27,195 ($21,611-$32,779)	$21,172 ($16,823-$24,738)	$48,377 ($39,230-$98,288)
Age Group			
<55	$31,125 ($23,730-$38,519)	$23,573 ($17,407-$32,976)	$57,566 ($47,246-$139,355)
55-64	$28,014 ($20,062-$35,965)	$18,095 ($13,919-$24,409)	$48,112 ($40,549-$101,176)
65+	$34,846 ($27,542-$42,151)	$26,103 ($21,309-$38,092)	$82,815 ($57,774-$98,288)
Collaborative Stage			
Stage III	$32,778 ($24,509-$41,046)	$25,530 ($18,095-$32,530)	$61,661 ($46,706-$194,171)
Stage IV	$30,207 ($24,959-$35,455)	$21,491 ($16,823-$24,738)	$68,661 ($48,651-$98,288)
Histology			
Adeno-carcinomas	$31,787 ($25,793-$37,781)	$21,910 ($18,655-$25,679)	$68,661 ($48,455-$101,176)
Large cell	$31,259 ($23,775-$38,743)	$24,287 ($14,212-$34,749)	$82,815 ($48,112-$98,288)
Squamous cell	$24,566 ($13,406-$35,725)	$19,144 ($9,731-$34,340)	$40,549 ($32,976-$88,838)
Smoking History			
Non-Smoker	$51,764 ($28,632-$74,897)	$28,294 ($18,762-$80,873)	$121,658 ($88,170-$185,370)
Smoker	$33,261 ($24,247-$42,275)	$23,345 ($15,350-$33,549)	$84,388 ($56,713-$194,171)
ex-Smoker	$24,415 ($19,889-$28,940)	$21,700 ($16,845-$30,050)	$44,280 ($36,731-$82,815)

Table 3. (Continued)

	Mean Cost (95% CI)	Median Cost (95% CI)	90th Cost (95% CI)
unknown	$26,831 ($20,955-$32,706)	$21,172 ($15,008-$27,556)	$48,642 ($40,549-$97,489)
1st Line Chemo Agents			
Platin-Gem	$32,684 ($26,103-$39,265)	$21,970 ($16,845-$30,608)	$84,942 ($55,776-$97,489)
Platin-Pax	$31,832 ($20,155-$43,509)	$23,633 ($17,087-$30,434)	$84,491 ($33,076-$139,355)
Platin-Vin	$25,049 ($18,044-$32,053)	$20,305 ($12,984-$32,976)	$56,713 ($38,122-$84,388)
none	$26,613 ($15,715-$37,510)	$15,542 ($8,923-$40,885)	$52,767 ($40,885-$70,324)
other	$38,029 ($10,940-$65,118)	$22,822 ($13,769-$47,246)	$48,651 ($47,246-$194,171)
Intended Treatment Line			
1	$26,613 ($15,715-$37,510)	$15,542 ($8,923-$40,885)	$52,767 ($40,885-$70,324)
2	$34,864 ($24,912-$44,816)	$21,433 ($14,212-$26,103)	$88,838 ($48,651-$185,370)
3	$28,416 ($23,975-$32,858)	$22,617 ($18,762-$29,091)	$55,788 ($46,706-$84,942)
4	$37,182 ($11,204-$63,160)	$30,437 ($13,276-$103,961)	$103,961 ($36,731-$103,961)
with Hospitalization			
No	$10,632 ($7,823-$13,441)	$8,836 ($6,629-$13,295)	$24,409 ($15,008-$33,076)
Yes	$34,980 ($29,995-$39,966)	$25,373 ($22,029-$31,018)	$82,815 ($55,800-$97,446)
with Hospital ER entry			
No	$27,500 ($21,171-$33,828)	$16,994 ($13,295-$22,029)	$70,324 ($47,834-$88,838)
Yes	$34,366 ($28,228-$40,504)	$26,431 ($22,376-$32,132)	$65,161 ($48,112-$98,288)
CCI Score Group			
CCI count = 1	$32,746 ($23,693-$41,800)	$21,239 ($15,228-$33,076)	$61,661 ($55,776-$194,171)
CCI count = 2	$33,474 ($26,803-$40,145)	$24,902 ($21,886-$32,530)	$84,439 ($47,246-$101,176)
CCI count = 3	$27,984 ($18,794-$37,173)	$19,450 ($13,525-$29,091)	$52,767 ($38,122-$139,355)
CCI count > 3	$12,527 ($6,139-$18,916)	$9,206 ($8,823-$13,958)	$25,613 ($11,474-$37,268)

For those in the 90th percentile of cost, Erlotinib cost \$65,307 (95% CI: \$48,513 - \$84,866). Total cost was higher for females (\$33,686, CI: \$27,169 – \$40,203) than males (\$26,644, 95% CI: \$21,264 - \$32,024). Hospitalization costs and prescriptions filled comprise more than 90% of total treatment costs with \$14,327.05 of costs going to hospital stays and \$14,497.01 going to drugs costs. We previously demonstrated that, with no cancer treatment after the last chemotherapy, the average cost per patients was \$13,539, and the average cost per patient-month was \$2,126, accounting for inflation. Hospital costs increased over this time as well: the base for CMG RIW (Resources Intensity Weight) increased from \$2,307 in 1997-1998 (10) to \$5,374 in 2008-09.

Several patterns can be observed in regards to cost by demographics. Men paid slightly more per week (\$1164) compared women (\$918). Individuals diagnosed with Stage IV (\$1033) paid slightly more per week as compared to individuals with Stage III (\$904). Smokers paid more per week (\$1145) compared to non-smokers (\$926), ex-smokers (\$901), and individuals with an unknown status (\$933). Individuals that were hospitalized (\$1083) paid over double per week compared to those without hospitalization (\$443). As comorbidity increased, so did the cost of treatment per week. For those with a CCI count greater than 3 (n = 10) cost was higher (\$1843) compared to those with one CCI count (\$883).

DISCUSSION

This study reports the treatment, outcomes, service utilization and associated costs of metastatic NSCLC patients who completed chemotherapy, and received Erlotinib as the second or third line treatment. The patient cohort for this study is small (n = 177), but allows for adequate comparison of costs association with various patient characteristics. The present study included an equal number of men and women, as well as smokers and non-smokers. As such, our investigation provides a wide range of information on costs. Our results suggested that patients that were currently smoking incurred higher costs per week compared to ex-smokers or non-smokers.

The principal strength of this study is that it is a population-based real cost analysis specifically addressing costs of Erlotnib in Manitoba, Canada. Most studies have examined cost effectiveness in Europe (26) and the United States (25), which are likely not representative of cost within the Canadian health care system. The present study includes all patients diagnosed with metastatic NSCLC who were approved for and used Erlotinib. While many studies have examined the cost effectiveness of the treatment of NSCLC patients, most have been undertaken in the context of clinical trials. In referring to economic evaluations, Coyle et al., stated that 'trials may be unsuitable for a number of reasons, such as inappropriate comparator, inappropriate choice of endpoints, atypical settings and treatment protocols, insufficient sample size for resource and cost variables and inadequate length of follow-up' (13, p.141). Others have also expressed concerns about the generalizability or external validity of studies associated with clinical trials (14-17).

The median survival time of our patients was 40.1 weeks from the date of approval for Erlotinib. Direct comparison with other published studies is hazardous as most of them are RCTs with strict patient inclusion criteria (18-20). However, it is reassuring that the median survival in this small cohort seems better or at least comparable. Our previous population-based study of no cancer treatment after chemotherapy found a survival of 17.8 weeks from the last cycle of chemotherapy. These two studies are not directly comparable, but the increase of 22.3 weeks in median survival found in this study indicates that the improved survival with Erlotinib seen in RCT can also be observed in population- based study.

The most notable difference between this study and our previous study (no cancer treatment after completion of chemotherapy) was that, in this study, there were only 1.5 hospitalizations per person and these accounted for approximately 45% of the health care costs, while in the previous study there were 1.9 hospitalizations per person accounting for 83% of total costs (10). We found clear benefits of introducing Erlotinib: increases in survival coupled with decreasing numbers of episodes of hospitalization. Even though quality of life was not assessed in this study, previous studies have determined Erlotinib to be more cost effective due to less costs related to management of side effects resulting in higher quality of life and less hospitalization (26).

The average cost per patient was $30,991 and average cost per patient-month was $3,314 from the date of last chemotherapy. Because health care costs vary across countries, it is difficult to compare costs across countries examining the cost of Erlotinib. However, the overall average cost fit within the CA$17,000 to CA$50,000 range of cost for Erlotinib in previous studies in Europe and the US (25, 26). Our earlier study [10] showed that the average cost per patient since date of last chemotherapy until death, prior to the introduction of Erlotinib, was $13,539 and the average cost per patient-month was $2,126. Cost-effectiveness analyses of Erlotinib have been published, mostly based on clinical trial results. Incremental cost-effectiveness ratio for Erlotinib treatment was $94,638 in 2007 Canadian dollars per life year gained, which was at the upper boundary of both Canadian and US thresholds historically accepted as cost-effective (22). Ramsey et al. (2008) reported that expenditures for all services increased for individuals receiving second- and third-line chemotherapy (21). We can consequently expect greater costs for treating NCSLC patients with the introduction of expensive lung cancer drugs. Our study has demonstrated that there is, in fact, an absolute increase in the total cost with the introduction of Erlotinib. However, this increase in average cost by $14,879 was accompanied by fewer hospital admissions per person and improved survival.

The majority of services that were utilized by the patients in this study were physician visits and prescriptions filled. One limitation of this study is that, since all the medical claims from the time of last chemotherapy were included, some of them may not be related to lung cancer. Pain and shortness of breath are symptoms experienced by the majority of late-stage lung cancer patients, which certainly contributed to the high use of narcotics. Erlotinib made up the largest portion of 3,160 prescriptions, followed by cardiovascular drugs. This may reflect the fact that lung cancer patients are generally elderly and smokers with associated high co-morbidities.

One of the cost effectiveness factors related to Erlotinib is the reduction in impactful side effects. Prior studies found that reduction in management of side effects between Erlotinib and chemo treatments as an important cost saving measure (26). While the present study did not compare Erlotinib to any other treatment, we did generate cost per week for patients. We observed higher costs between patients that were hospitalized and hospitalized with ER visits. Because of the relatively small sample size, we were unable to examine the characteristics of individuals that did or did not seek hospital visits. Future research should aim to examine what care demographics relate to decreased likelihood of emergency hospitalization.

Our study adds to this existing literature, because we evaluated Erlotinib in a real-world setting. The costs experienced by patients in a real-world setting are likely to be greater than costs incurred in clinical trials, in which the patient population is usually more tightly selected. Very recently, two studies in British Columbia evaluated the cost-effectiveness of Erlotinib in a real-world setting (23, 24). They suggested that Erlotinib may be a cost-effective treatment as a third-line agent, but not as a second-line agent, compared to all treatment received within the health care system from end of second line treatment to death or censoring. Cromwell et al. (24) have estimated the cost effectiveness of Erlotinib comparing the historical control and found that the mean incremental cost (ICER) was around $36, 000 per year of life gained.

Our study also showed a positive comparative analysis, where the comparison is made between patients who received no further cancer treatment after completion of chemotherapy and those who received Erlotinib. We did not estimate ICER using the historical control, however the comparative results suggest the estimation will be very close to what was estimated by Cromwell et al. (24).

This study is neither designed to compare the survival nor to calculate the cost effectiveness of Erlotinib. Additionally, the present study did not compare how the cost of Erlotinib to other second line agents such as docetaxel and pemetrexed, as well as cost effectiveness for individuals with EGFR wild type gene. Currently, Erlotinib is the standard of care for metastatic NSCLC as a second or third line agent and thus it will not be possible to get a similar study cohort without the treatment. Acknowledging the limitation of the study, the results have indicated that, while there is an increase in health care cost with the introduction of Erlotinib, this is accompanied by improved survival and a reduction in the number of hospital admissions, and consequently an improvement in quality of life, in the real world setting.

REFERENCES

[1] Parkin DM. Global cancer statistics in the year 2000. Lancet Oncol 2001;2:533–43.

[2] Sher T, Dy W, Adjei AA. Small cell lung cancer. Mayo Clin Proc 2008 83:355–67.

[3] Travis WD, Travis LB, Devera SS. Lung cancer. Cancer 1995;75:191–202.

[4] Franeschi S, Bidoli E, The epidemiology of lung cancer. Ann Oncol 1999;10:S3–S6.

[5] Pitz MW, Musto G, Demers A, Kliewer EV, Navaratnam S. 20 year population based analysis of treatment and survival with non-small cell lung cancer in Manitoba, Canada: combination of registry and administrative data. J Thorac Oncol 2009;4(4):492-8.

[6] Coleman MP, Forman D, Bryant H, Butler J, Rachet B, Maringe C, et al. Cancer survival in Australia, Canada, Denmark, Norway, Sweden, and the UK, 1995-2007 (the International Cancer Benchmarking Partnership): An analysis of population-based cancer registry data. Lancet 2011;377(9760):127-38.

[7] Stinchcombe TE, Lee CB, Socinski MA. Current approaches to advanced stage non-small cell lung cancer: first line therapy in patients with good functional status. Clin Lung Cancer 2006;4(7):S111–7.

[8] Felip E, Rosell R. Pemetrexed as second-line therapy for advanced non-small cell lung cancer (NSCLC). Ther Clin Risk Manage 2008;4:579–85.

[9] Shepherd FA, Pereira JR, Ciuleanu T, Tan EH, Hirsh V, Thongprasert S, et al. Erlotinib in previously treated non-small cell lung cancer. N Engl J Med 2005;353(2):123–32.

[10] Navaratnam S, Kliewer EV, Butler J, Demers AA, Musto G, Badiani K. Population-based patterns and cost of management of metastatic non-small cell lung cancer after completion of chemotherapy until death. Lung Cancer 2010;70(1):110-5.

[11] Sisler J, Seo B, Katz A, Shu E, Chateau D, Czaykowski P, et al. Concordance with ASCO guidelines for surveillance after colorectal cancer treatment: A population-based analysis. J Oncol Pract 2012;8(4):e69-79. doi: 10.1200/JOP. 2011.000396.

[12] Roos LL, Brownell M, Lix L, Roos NP, Walld R, MacWilliam L. From health research to social research: Privacy, methods, approaches. Soc Sci Med 2008;66(1):117-29.

[13] Coyle D, Davies L, Drummond MF. Emerging issues in designing economic evaluations alongside clinical trials. Int J Technol Assess Health Care 1998;14:135-44.

[14] Quoix E, Finkelstein H, Wolkove N, Kreisman H. Treatment of small-cell lung cancer on protocol: potential bias of results. J Clin Oncol 1986;4(9):1314-20.

[15] Watkin SW, Hayhurst GK, Green JA. Time trends in the outcome of lung cancer management: a study of 9,090 cases diagnosed in the Mersey Region, 1974-86. Br J Cancer 1990;61:590-6.

[16] Leighl NB, Shepherd FA, Kwong R, Burkes RL, Feld R, Goodwin PJ. Economic analysis of the TAX 317 trial: docetaxel versus best supportive care as second-line therapy of advanced non-small cell lung cancer. J Clin Oncol 2002;20(5):1344-52.

[17] Ramsey SD, Moinpour CM, Lovato LC, Crowley JJ, Grevstad P, Presant CA, et al. Economic analysis of vinorelbine plus cisplatin versus paclitaxel plus carboplatin for advanced non-small-cell lung cancer. J Nat Cancer Inst 2002;94(4):291-7.

[18] Hanna N, Shepherd F, Fossella FV, Pereira JR, De Marinis F, von Pawel J, et al. Randomized phase III trial of pemetrexed versus docetaxel in patients with non-small-cell lung cancer previously treated with chemotherapy. J Clin Oncol 2004;22(9):1589-97.

[19] Smit EF, Mattson K, von Pawel J, Manegold C, Clarke S, Postmus PE. ALIMTA (pemetrexed disodium) as second-line treatment of non-small-cell lung cancer: A Phase II study. Ann Oncol 2003;14(3):455-60.

[20] Ng R, Loreto M, Lee R, Leighl NB. Brief report: Retrospective review of efficacy of erlotinib or gefitinib compared to docetaxel as subsequent line therapy in advanced non-small-cell lung cancer (NSCLC) following failure of platinum-based chemotherapy. Lung Cancer 2008;61(2):262-5.

[21] Ramsey SD, Martins RG, Blough DK, Tock LS, Lubeck D, Reyes CM. Second-line and third-line chemotherapy for lung cancer: Use and cost. Am J Manag Care 2008;14(5): 297-306.

[22] Bradbury PA, Tu D, Seymour L, Isogai PK, Zhu L, Ng R, et al. Economic analysis: Randomized placebo-controlled clinical trial of erlotinib in advanced non–small cell lung cancer. J Natl Cancer Inst 2010;102(5):298-306.

[23] Cromwell I, Melosky B, van der Hoeck K, Melosky B, Peacock S. Erlotinib or docetaxel for 2nd line treatment for non-small cell lung cancer: A real world cost-effectiveness analysis. J Thorac Oncol 2011;6(12):2097-103.

[24] Cromwell I, van der Hoeck K, Malfair Taylor SC, Melosky B, Peacock S. Erlotinib or best supportive care for third-line treatment of advanced non-small-cell lung cancer: A real-world cost-effectiveness analysis. Lung Cancer 2012;76(3):472-7.

[25] Carlson JJ, Reyes C, Oestreicher N, Lubeck D, Ramsey SD, Veenstra DL. Comparative clinical and economic outcomes of treatments for refractory non-small cell lung cancer (NSCLC). Lung Cancer 2008;61(3):405-15.

[26] Lewis G, Peake M, Aultman R, Gyldmark M, Morlotti L, Creeden J, et al. Cost-effectiveness of erlotinib versus docetaxel for second-line treatment of advanced non –small-cell lung cancer in the United Kingdom. J Int Med Res 2010;38:9–21.

In: Clinical Oncology
Editors: Ariel Tenenbaum et al.
ISBN: 978-1-53617-933-0

Chapter 15

EARLY ONCOLOGY REHABILITATION (EOR) FOR LYMPHOMA PATIENTS: A REVIEW OF FUNCTIONAL OUTCOMES AND INPATIENT REHABILITATION PILOT PROGRAM IN SINGAPORE GENERAL HOSPITAL (SGH)

Saw H Mar**, Tan Y Leng, Jiang Yan,
Aung M Oo, Bok C Wai and Ng Y Sien
Department of Rehabilitation Medicine,
Department of Quality Management, Department of Nursing Division,
Singapore General Hospital, Singapore

* Corresponding Author: Saw Hay Mar, MBBS, MRCP, FAMS, Associate Consultant, Department of Rehabilitation Medicine, Singapore General Hospital, Outram Road, 169608 Singapore. E-mail: saw.hay.mar@singhealth.com.sg.

Abstract

Lymphoma is one of the top ten cancers in Singapore. Functional impairments of lymphoma patients during treatments for underlying pathology increase the demand for initiation of early rehabilitation program. This chapter aims to review demographics data and short term functional outcomes of lymphoma subjects with early oncology rehabilitation (EOR) pilot program. Methods: Rehabilitation Medicine and Medical Oncology Departments started pilot program with weekly multidisciplinary team meeting (MDM) to offer them EOR service under either inpatient rehabilitation team (IRT) or primary oncology team (OCT). Forty-seven lymphoma patients completed the program. Our outcome measures included Functional Independence Measure (FIM), length of stay (LOS) and ambulatory distance at the point of discharge. Results: The IRT group had higher number of patients with cognitive issue (57.9%) than the OCT group (28.6%). None of the patients in the IRT and 21.4% in the OCT groups were ADL-independent ($p = 0.035$) at first MDM. Median cognitive FIM on admission for the IRT cohort was lower than OCT cohort ($p = 0.004$). Median total LOS in the IRT and OCT groups was (36 days vs 13 days, $p <0.005$), and median acute LOS in the former and latter (17 days vs 13 days, $p =0.017$). Motor FIM gain of both IRT and OCT groups was significant ($p =0.002$ vs $p = 0.008$). Both cohorts reported improvement in ambulatory distance ($p <0.001$ vs $p = 0.001$). Conclusion: Reviewing the characteristic and functional outcomes of our program supports the feasibility of multidisciplinary approach rehabilitation in acute medical setting.

Introduction

Recent advances in cancer screening, early detection and treatments have resulted in increasing number of cancer survivors. The American Cancer Society reported that as of 1st January 2016, there were more than 15.5 million cancer survivors in US and the number is estimated to rise further up to nearly 20.3 million by 2026 (1). Among cancer subgroups, it is estimated to have 81,080 newly diagnosed cases of lymphoma in 2016 in America (2). In Singapore, according to data from Singapore Cancer Registry dated 2010 to 2014, lymphoma is the fifth and sixth most common cause of cancer in males and females with 2023 and 1410 cases respectively (3). Due to aggressive nature of the disease, lymphoma patients usually require intensive treatments with multiple regimes such as chemotherapy, radiotherapy, surgery, transplant, biologic therapy and sometimes combination of those treatments. These treatments often necessitate a considerable length of hospital stay which led to numerous adverse functional outcomes including physical deconditioning, cognitive impairments, fatigue, depression, reduced quality of life (QoL), pain and bone mass loss (4). As rehabilitation can potentially reverse poor physical functional outcomes in cancer patients, it has been perceived as a very important and integral part of comprehensive cancer management (5-8). According to World Health Organization (WHO) world report on disability, rehabilitation has been defined as a set of measures that assist individuals who experience or are likely to experience disability to achieve and maintain optimal functioning in interaction with their environments (9).

In Singapore General Hospital (SGH), well established rehabilitation programs for stroke, hip fracture, spinal cord injury and amputation exist with clinical pathways facilitating workflow and early initiation of rehabilitation. However, there was no formal oncology rehabilitation pathway due to complexity of cancer treatment regime and limited understanding of oncology rehabilitation (10). As survival improves and cancer becomes a chronic condition, many oncological patients require rehabilitation services to maintain their physical and psychological well beings (11-16). Prior to May 2015, cancer patients who required inpatient rehabilitation were referred to SGH Department of Rehabilitation Medicine through on-call specialist consultation service. These referrals were often ad-hoc without multidisciplinary approaches. Challenges with these ad-hoc referrals were delay in prompt identification of impairments by primary teams, lack of holistic communication between therapists, rehabilitation physicians, nurses and oncologists and often led to delay in referral to rehabilitation team and hence initiation of exercises. As time passes, physicians and members of the Allied Health acknowledged the necessity to initiate an early rehabilitation program to identify impairments and administer effective cancer exercise programs. The SGH Department of

Rehabilitation Medicine formulated a concept involving oncologists, rehabilitation physicians, nurses and members of the Allied Health to create an inpatient oncology rehabilitation program for cancer patients to commence early rehabilitation therapy to improve their functional outcomes. In May 2015, Rehabilitation Medicine and Medical Oncology Departments started a pilot collaboration program with weekly multidisciplinary team meeting (MDM) for lymphoma cancer sub-group and offered them early oncology rehabilitation (EOR) service under either inpatient rehabilitation team (IRT) or oncology team (OCT) at SGH.

In this study, we aim to review a one-year data from this pilot collaboration. Besides reviewing the demographics of lymphoma patients undergoing early oncology rehabilitation pilot program, this study i) compares short term functional outcomes of lymphoma patients between two groups, early oncology rehabilitation program under inpatient rehabilitation team (IRT) vs under primary oncology team (OCT); ii) highlights the strengths and weaknesses of the pilot program; and iii) comment on the feasibility of early rehabilitation program under oncology team co-managed by rehabilitation physician led weekly MDM and workflow system.

OUR STUDY

The team members of pilot program comprise of the Allied Health (physiotherapist, occupational therapists, speech and language therapist, medical social worker and dietician), nurses, rehabilitation physicians and oncologists. The aim of the MDM was to highlight functional goals and strategize pragmatic rehabilitation programs to assist the individual lymphoma patients with rehabilitation needs. Discussion was led by rehabilitation physician and oncologist with charting of functional outcomes using Functional Independence Measure (FIM). Rehabilitation issues and needs for lymphoma patients were divided into two main domains, namely, physical aspects and psychosocial aspects as per check list form shown in Figure 1. The check list assessment was conducted by a medical officer or resident nurse upon the first day of admission to oncology unit for every lymphoma patient. If a lymphoma patient had two or more rehabilitation issues from the check list, the case would be brought up for further detailed discussion during MDM. Rehabilitation specialist reviewed the details of the patients' medical conditions and assessment included diagnosis, staging, investigations, treatment regime, prognosis of cancer, premorbid functional status and current functional level and patient's motivation. The oncologist clarified questions related to cancer and its treatment raised by MDM team members to assist in the decision making process of selecting suitable lymphoma patients for inpatient rehabilitation.

The EOR program facilities comprised of indoor walking tracks, aerobic and strength training machines, free weighs, transfer and ambulation assistive devices and assessment to functional training. The Physiotherapist, Occupational therapist and Speech and Language therapists review the patients 3 to 5 times a week, 30 to 45 min per each session as duration of the session was catered to individual endurance level. Each patient was given individualized exercise program which consists of cardiovascular training, resistance training or both. If patients were not well or unstable during therapy, therapists stopped the session and immediately informed primary team doctors to access for suitability of continuation of therapy. The therapists reported baseline functional assessment level as well as patients' and families' goals at the start of program. They also reported daily detail training program which included intensity, duration, frequency, type of exercises and progress. Dietitian reviewed the patients and provided nutritional counseling and diet schedules upon admission followed by weekly reviews. The significance of this program was continuation of early rehabilitation despite the participants had ongoing acute medical treatments such as chemotherapy, radiotherapy for underlying disease and or acute medical issues such as electrolytes imbalances and sepsis but not requiring closer monitoring.

Name of Patient: **NRIC:** **Date of Birth:** **Ward/Bed:**			
No.	Symptoms	Tick	Comment
Physical Aspects			
1	Fatigue and poor endurance		
2	Weakness of upper limbs/lower limbs		
3	Difficulties in ambulation/Balance/Fall issues		
4	Difficulties in ADL		
5	Cognitive issues		
6	Speech and language disorders/Swallowing disorders		
7	Bowel and bladder issues (constipation, retention of urine, high PVRU, failed TOC)		
8	Poor nutrition		
9	If patient requires chest physiotherapy/shortness of breath during activity		
Psychosocial Aspects			
1	Practical aspects of care and arrangements needed (home modification and equipment prescription)		
2	Caregiver training/Care giver issues/Care giver distress		
3	Need of financial assistance		
4	Motivation Issues		

Abbreviation: ADL, Activities of daily livings; PVRU, Post void residual urine; TOC, Trial of catheter.

Figure 1. Check List for Oncology Rehabilitation Multidisciplinary Team Meeting and Referral.

Patient selection

Inclusion criteria to EOR were 1) patients who had ≥ 2 rehabilitation issues in the check list form, 2) stable vital signs (blood pressure > 90/60 mmHg, heart rate > 60/min and < 120/min, oxygen saturation ≥ 95% on room air or oxygen requirement not more than 2L/min), 3) haemoglobin ≥ 8g/dl, (4) absolute neutrophil count (ANC) ≥ 0.5x 19^9/L, 5) platelet counts ≥ 30,000x10^9/L, 6) age ≥ 21 years and 7) patients who agreed to enroll into the program. For patients who were suitable for EOR program, the MDM team members made decision about maintaining some lymphoma patients under oncology team (OCT) vs. transferring under inpatient rehabilitation team (IRT) based on their cancer and other medical treatment duration. For instance, if patients require substantial amount of time to complete inpatient cancer treatment or antibiotic regimes, decision was made to be taken over by IRT.

Exclusion criteria were 1) unstable vital sings (BP < 90/60, HR < 60/min or >120/min, oxygen saturation < 95% despite intranasal oxygen supplement 2L/min), 2) haemoglobin < 8g/dl, 3) absolute neutrophil count (ANC) < 0.5x 19^9/L,(4) platelet counts < 30,000x10^9/L, 5) atrial fibrillation, 6) < 5 day post myocardial infarct (AMI), 7) age < 21 years 8) patients who did not agree to participate in the EOR and 9) if their rehabilitation issues can be resolved within a short period of time (i.e., within < 5 days) while in the oncology unit. Examples of these rehabilitation issues include equipment prescription, home modification advice, financial assistance for rehabilitation equipment and choice of outpatient rehabilitation services after discharge. Patients who were excluded from EOR still continue to receive ward level therapy until they were discharged from the oncology ward.

Data collection and outcome measures

We conducted retrospective data review of fifty-four lymphoma patients who received EOR program between May 2015 and April 2016. The clinical data of these lymphoma patients were brought up for the MDM discussion. Clinical information were recorded under the hospital electronic referral system and information was password protected. We collected demographic data such as age, gender, ethnicity, employment status at the point of admission and number of co-morbidities at the point of hospital admission. In terms of the oncology disease, information such as lymphoma with central nervous system involvement or spinal cord involvement was included. The reason for hospital admission for every lymphoma patient was also evaluated, i.e., lymphoma patients who were admitted for treatment of underlying oncological condition or admission due to complications from the treatments.

In our EOR program, patients' short term functional outcome measure was assessed by functional independence measures (FIM score). FIM is widely used rehabilitation scale to assess physical and cognitive impairments and it focuses on the level of the burden of care (17, 18). The scales consists of 13 items of physical and 5 items of cognitive domains, with each item scores from a scale of 1 to 7, 1 represents total dependence and 7 indicates complete independence. The admission and discharge FIM scores were documented by the oncology-rehabilitation MDM team members. FIM scoring at first MDM discussion was documented as admission FIM score. We also recorded ambulatory distance (in meters) in all these patients. Ambulatory distance is defined as the maximum ambulatory distance a patient can ambulate with or without the use of walking aid. Other outcome measures such as total, acute and rehabilitation length of stay (LOS), their activities of daily livings (ADL), ambulation status and complications were also recorded. In term of LOS, total LOS (TLOS) refers to length of stay from the first day of acute admission to discharge, acute LOS (ALOS) means from the first day of acute admission until transfer under rehabilitation team and rehabilitation LOS (RLOS) represents number of days patients spent after taken over under rehabilitation team. If the patient was not taken over under rehabilitation team, then, their acute LOS was same as total LOS.

Statistical analysis

Statistical analysis was done using Statistical Package for Social Sciences (SPSS) software version 20. Statistical significance was reported in 2-tailed and determined at P values <0.05. Categorical data are shown in number (%), continuous data are shown in median (range) Mann-Whitney U test for continuous variables and Fisher's exact test for categorical variables. Univariate analysis of FIM score and ambulatory distance were carried out using Wilcoxon Sign Rank test.

FINDINGS

Over a period of twelve months from May 2015 to April 2016, fifty-four patients met criteria for early oncology rehabilitation. Seven patients were excluded from the study due to mortality on the same admission. Table 1 summarizes the baseline characteristic of the study patients. For the forty-seven patients remained in the study, nineteen received early oncology rehabilitation program under inpatient rehabilitation team (IRT) while the rest of the twenty-eight were under primary oncology team (OCT). In terms of demographic data, the median age of patients between two groups was 67.0 years for the IRT and 66.5 years for OCT cohorts respectively. The majority of patients were Chinese in both groups (IRT 68.4%, n=13 and OCT 67.9%, n=19) and male patients formed the majority in the IRT group than their male counterpart in OCT group (IRT 68.4%, n= 13 and OCT 46.4%, n=13). Most of the patients in both IRT and OCT cohorts had comorbidities (IRT 78.9%, n=15 and OCT 85.7%, n=24) of which 15.8% (n=3) of the IRT group had 3 or more comorbidities compared to 21.4% (n=6) in the OCT. Most of the patients in study population were not employed at the time of admission with only 15.8% (n=3) being employed in the IRT group and 39.3% (n=11) in the OCT group. There was no statistical significance between the median age, gender, ethnicity, employment status at the point of hospital admission and the number of existing co-morbidities of the two cohorts.

For the oncological condition, central nervous system(CNS) and spinal cord involvement(SC) were similar in IRT group and OCT group (CNS: IRT 47.7% (n=9) and OCT 35.7% (n=10); SC: IRT 21.1% (n=4) and OCT 14.3% (n=4) respectively). Notably, there were more patients with complication related admission in the OCT cohort than the IRT group (OCT 39.3%, n=11 and IRT 26.3%, n=5). In terms of rehabilitation issues, the IRT group had higher number of patients with cognitive issue (57.9%, n=11) than the OCT group (28.6%, n=8).

Table 1. Baseline characteristics of study population

	Lymphoma Patients		
	IRT	OCT	*P* value
	N = 19	N = 28	
Age	67.0 (37.0)	66.5 (62.0)	0.515
Male	13 (68.4)	13 (46.4)	0.117
Chinese	13 (68.4)	19 (67.9)	0.612
Employment (Y)	3 (15.8)	11 (39.3)	0.078
CNS involvement	9 (47.7)	10 (35.7)	0.309
Spinal Cord involvement	4 (21.1)	4 (14.3)	0.411
Reason for admission			0.274
Complication	5 (26.3)	11 (39.3)	
Oncology treatment	14 (73.7)	17 (60.7)	
Rehabilitation issues			
Mobility	19 (100)	27 (96.4)	0.596
Cognitive	11 (57.9)	8 (28.6)	0.044
Comorbidity	15 (78.9)	24 (85.7)	0.411
3 or more comorbidities	3 (15.8)	6 (21.4)	0.465
History of cancer	7 (36.8)	10 (35.7)	0.589

Categorical data are shown in number (%), continuous data are shown in median (range).
Mann-Whitney U test for continuous variables and Fisher's exact test for categorical variables.
Abbreviation: IRT, Inpatient rehabilitation team; OCT, Oncology team; CNS, Central nervous system.

There was no statistical significant difference in their baseline premorbid ADL, ambulation status and gait aid requirement for the two groups. At the point of first rehabilitation review, i.e., first MDM, there was statistical difference in their ADL status in IRT group compared to OCT group. None of the patients in the IRT group were ADL-independent which is a contrast with the OCT group where 21.4% (n=6) of lymphoma patients were ADL-independent ($p = 0.035$). Moreover, more patients in the IRT group showed more gait aid requirement than their OCT counterpart (89.5% vs 60.7%, $p= 0.030$). There was also significant differences in LOS, the median TLOS in IRT and OCT groups (36 days vs 13 days, $p <0.005$), and median ALOS in the former and latter (17 days vs 13 days, $p =0.017$). At the point of hospital discharge, neither of the two groups showed superiority in terms of ADL independency, independence in ambulation status and gait aid requirement.

The median motor FIM on admission and discharge were similar for both groups. However, the median FIM (cognitive) admission for the IRT group was much lower than OCT group (19 vs 33, p = 0.004). At the point of discharge, there was no statistically significance difference for median cognitive FIM scores between these two groups. In addition, the admission and discharge ambulation distance and complications were similar in both groups.

Table 2. Rehabilitation outcomes compare analysis

	Lymphoma Patients		
	IRT	OCT	*P* value
	N = 19	N = 28	
ADL(Independent)			
Pre morbid	14 (73.7)	20 (71.4)	0.568
Frist MDM	0 (0.0)	6 (21.4)	0.035
Discharge	1 (5.3)	7 (25.0)	0.081
Gait aid			
Admission	8 (42.1)	9 (32.1)	0.347
First MDM	17 (89.5)	17 (60.7)	0.030
Discharge	11 (57.9)	16 (57.1)	0.599
Ambulation (Independent)			
Pre morbid	14 (73.7)	23 (82.1)	0.366
First MDM	2 (10.5)	7 (25.0)	0.197
Discharge	5 (26.3)	8 (28.6)	0.568
Ambulatory Distance (Meters)			
Admission	6.0 (80.0)	9.0 (100.0)	0.277
Discharge	40.0 (150.0)	20.0 (200.0)	0.154
FIM (Motor)			
Admission	39.0 (40.0)	41.0 (61.0)	0.340
Discharge	50.0 (61.0)	46.0 (74.0)	0.656
FIM (Cognitive)			
Admission	19.0 (28.0)	33.0 (25.0)	0.004
Discharge	25.0 (28.0)	32.5 (27.0)	0.070
Acute LOS (days)	17.0 (120.0)	13.0 (76.0)	0.017
Total LOS (days)	36.0 (118.0)	13.0 (76.0)	0.000
Rehab LOS (days)	14.0 (24.0)	NA	
Complications (any)	14 (73.7)	21 (75.0)	0.590

Categorical data are shown in number (%), continuous data are shown in median (range).
Mann-Whitney U test for continuous variables and Fisher's exact test for categorical variables.
Abbreviation: ADL, Activities of daily living; MDM, Multidisciplinary team meeting; LOS, Length of stay.

Using Wilcoxon Signed Rank Test, we further sub-analyzed the individual group for improvements in their admission and discharge median FIM score and ambulatory distance. Patients in IRT who received early oncology rehabilitation program had significant improvement in motor FIM gain, i.e., the difference between FIM on discharge and admission (p =0.002). Likewise, the FIM gain in the OCT cohort was statistically significant (p = 0.008). In contrast, cognitive FIM score in both groups had no improvement in both groups, admission and discharge cognitive FIM. Both cohorts also reported significant improvement in ambulatory distance (IRT, p<0.001; OCT, p=0.001).

Table 3. Comparison of rehabilitation outcomes between IRT and OCT on admission and discharge

	Admission	Discharge	***P value**
Ambulatory Distance (Meters)			
IRT	6.0 (80.0)	40.0 (150.0)	<0.001
OCT	9.0 (100.0)	20.0 (200.0)	0.001
FIM (Motor)			
IRT	39.0 (40.0)	50.0 (61.0)	0.002
OCT	41.0 (61.0)	46.0 (74.0)	0.008
FIM (Cognitive)			
IRT	19.0 (28.0)	25.0 (28.0)	0.102
OCT	33.0 (25.0)	32.5 (27.0)	0.547

Continuous data are shown in median (range).

*Wilcoxon Sign Rank test.

Abbreviation: IRT, Inpatient rehabilitation team; OCT, Oncology team; FIM, Functional independence measure.

DISCUSSION

National Cancer Centre Singapore (NCCS) is the largest cancer center in Singapore, located within SGH campus and it provides unique oncology service with a wide range of cancer care, including medical management and rehabilitation of complex cancer patients. However, there seems to be limited formal cancer rehabilitation program in Singapore. Study by Tay et al. (10) suggested better cancer rehabilitation programs should be structured and refined. Previous studies showed that reported rates of physical impairment and disability in cancer survivors are high as a result of their cancer and or its treatment resulting limitation in daily activities and reduction of quality of life (7, 19, 20). As rehabilitation interventions can ameliorate physical and cognitive impairments and optimize functional outcomes, there is a growing need to collaborate between oncologist, rehabilitation physicians and Allied Health personnel. This pilot study formulates early inpatient rehabilitation program within Singapore National Cancer Center and is the first ever early oncology rehabilitation program locally.

Our study sample consisted of fifty-four lymphoma patients, of which, forty-seven patients completed early rehabilitation program. The median age of patients in our study is similar to the lymphoma patients in UK's population based study (21). Literatures supported that most lymphoid neoplasm often occur more in males than female, likewise, we had more male than female in our cohort (21, 22). Most of the patients in both IRT and OCT cohorts had underlying comorbidities which might affect health outcomes and functional capacity negatively after cancer diagnosis and its treatment (23, 24).

In our findings, key difference in patients under IRT compared to OCT were all dependent in ADLs, requiring more gait aids, rehabilitation issues with more cognitively impairment and lower FIM score upon first MDM consultation. This difference could be due to the selection process during MDM whereby those lymphoma patients who were more severely impaired were selected under inpatient rehabilitation team while those who were physically less dependent patients were discharged home directly from the oncology team after rehabilitation.

On further analysis on length of stay (LOS), both median total and acute LOS of the patients under IRT was significantly longer, possibly due to lower participation in rehabilitation and increased care needs in this cognitively more impaired group. The previous evidences similarly suggest that chemotherapy-related cognitive impairment has been observed in cancer patients with variable reports of impairment in memory, attention, concentration, executive function, processing speed, and visual-spatial skills. Likewise, cognitive dysfunction may complicate cancer or its treatment to the extent that basic function is undermined (25-27).

We compared the effect of early rehabilitation on functional outcomes of the two groups by using ambulation distance and FIM score. In rehabilitation, one of the goals is to encourage early mobility at least within the home (28). Our result revealed that both groups achieved significant improvement in ambulation distance after rehabilitation program. Their admission and discharge motor FIM were similar between IRT and OCT group, whereas, significant lower admission cognitive FIM in the former. Nonetheless, discharge cognitive FIM was comparable between two groups, suggested that implementation of early rehabilitation was worthwhile in cancer patients in acute clinical setting. In addition, these findings demonstrated that similar accomplishments in functional outcomes were met even if rehabilitation was carried out under oncology team with availability of opinions from rehabilitation multidisciplinary team. It is an important finding that enlisting the cooperation of the oncology team staffs together with rehabilitation team in the multidisciplinary team discussion can potentially value add rehabilitation practices for cancer patients. This finding supports our review on the feasibility of conducting early rehabilitation program under oncology team with rehabilitation physician led weekly MDM without the need for inpatient transfer from oncology team to the inpatient rehabilitation team.

We also sub-analyzed FIM and ambulatory distance of individual group. From admission to discharge, motor FIM scores improved 11 points and the median ambulatory distance improved 34 meters in the patients under rehabilitation team. That finding was encouraging, as it suggests rehabilitation under physiatrist led program could be translated into lower burden of care. FIM motor under OCT group also had improvement upon discharge with 5 points. On the other hand, none of the group attained statistically significant improvement in cognitive FIM scores. These data highlights to the fact that cognitive dysfunctions in lymphoma patients are enormous and their cognitive relearning may be slower. This may explain the significant increase in TLOS in the more cognitively impaired patients group in our program. It also underlines the importance of focused cognitive rehabilitation in cancer survivors to improve attention abilities and overall quality of life (29, 30).

This EOR program has several strengths. Our pilot program is the very first collaboration between the oncologist, rehabilitation physician, allied health services and nurses in an inpatient tertiary hospital setting. This program extends rehabilitation consultation to those lymphoma patients who remain in the oncology ward. In the local setting, comprehensive programs with tracking of rehabilitation functional outcome measures are usually carried out when patients are transferred under the care of the inpatient rehabilitation team from the oncology team. With increasing cancer population with rehabilitation needs, this new pilot program goes one step ahead of the conventional way of inpatient rehabilitation by early review and offering rehabilitation consultation opinion than the previously practiced ad-hoc referrals from the oncology team. Secondly, the EOR program has a multidisciplinary team approach where oncologists participate in the discussion of lymphoma patients. This would facilitate the rehabilitation team to understand the oncological condition better. Thirdly, our program is the first to explore early oncological rehabilitation in acute medical setting with lymphoma patients. These patients often have challenging oncology treatment, complicated medical issues related to the lymphoma disease and become deconditioned. Early mobilization, prevention of medical complications and screening of cognitive impairments in the oncology ward would ensure that none of the lymphoma patients in the oncology ward are omitted from rehabilitation care.

Another purpose of this EOR program review is to give health care providers a better understanding of the characteristics and the short term outcomes of the lymphoma patients in SGH. By reviewing the one year data, a comparison of short term functional outcomes in individuals who remained under the primary oncology team and those whose care was taken under the inpatient rehabilitation team would help healthcare providers to re-evaluate the current operational workflow of transferring patient from oncology department to the rehabilitation department. From the pilot study, the OCT group continues to make functional progress in terms of FIM and ambulation distance implying that a collaborative approach with a multidisciplinary practice might be useful. Moreover, the unique learning experience from this pilot program may be the platform to consider the expansion of early rehabilitation collaborative program for other oncology subgroups.

Our study has several limitations. Firstly, number of cancer population in this pilot program is small. Secondly, the study was conducted on lymphoma cancer sub-group only and therefore it is difficult to extrapolate results of this study to oncology patients at large. Moreover, rehabilitation focus should be on impairments driven rather than specific disease diagnosis. Lastly, there is lack of follow-up study on the longer term functional outcomes of the IRT and OCT cohorts after discharge. Apart from cognitive FIM score, other cognitive assessment scores of lymphoma patients are lacking in this study, hence it is difficult to conclude if any central nervous system involvement has significant impact on the FIM score gains.

CONCLUSION

In conclusion, this pilot program reviews the characteristic and short term functional outcomes of lymphoma patients who undergo early oncology rehabilitation. The findings from the pilot program supports the feasibility of changing the traditional work flow process from interdisciplinary to multidisciplinary approach might facilitate the overall rehabilitative care of lymphoma patients in a tertiary hospital. Further rehabilitation studies involving the entire oncology population should be considered to determine the efficacy of early oncology rehabilitation in acute clinical setting.

ACKNOWLEDGMENTS

The authors would like to express our deep gratitude to all multidisciplinary team meeting members, especially the nurses and allied health personnel from Singapore General Hospital Oncology ward, for their active involvements and support in this pilot program.

REFERENCES

[1] Cancer treatment and survivorship facts and figures 2016-2017. URL: http://www.cancer.org/acs/groups/content/@research/documents/document/acspc-048074.pdf.

[2] Cancer facts and figures 2016, American cancer society. URL: http://www.cancer.org/acs/groups/content/@research/documents/document/acspc-047079.pdf.

[3] Singapore cancer registry interim annual report trends in cancer incidence in Singapore: 2010-2014. URL: https://www.nrdo.gov.sg/.

[4] Courneya KS, Friedenreich CM. Framework PEACE: an organizational model for examining physical exercise across the cancer experience. Ann Behav Med 2001;23(4): 263–72.

[5] van Zutphen M, Winkels RM, van Duijnhoven FJ, van Harten-Gerritsen SA, Kok DE, van Duijvendijk, et al. An increase in physical activity after colorectal surgery is associated with improved recovery of physical functioning: a prospective cohort study. BMC Cancer 2017;17:74.

[6] Sloan JA, Cheville AL, Lui H, Novotny PJ, Wampfler JA, Yolanda I. Garces, et al. Impact of self-reported physical activity and health promotion behaviors on lung cancer survivorship. Health Quality Life Outcomes 2016;14:66.

[7] Lehmann JF, Delisa JA, Warren CG. Cancer rehabilitation: assessment of need, development, and evaluation of a model of care: Arch Phys Med Rehabil 1978;59(9): 410-9.

[8] Silver JK, Baima J, Mayer RS. Impairment-driven cancer rehabilitation: an essential component of quality care and survivorship. CA Cancer J Clin 2013;63(5):295-317.

[9] World Health Organization: WHO guidelines on health related rehabilitation. Geneva: World Health Organization, 2011. URL: www.who.int/disabilities/en/.

[10] Tay SS, Ng YS, Lim AC. Functional outcomes of cancer patients in an inpatient rehabilitation setting. Ann Acad Med Singapore 2009;38:197-201.

[11] McEwen S. Consensus recommendations for cancer rehab: research and education priorities. Curr Oncol 2013;20:64-9.

[12] Cole RP, Scialla SJ, Bednarz L. Functional recovery in cancer rehabilitation. Arch Phys Med Rehabil 2000;81:623-7.

[13] Wiskemann J, Dreger P, Schwerdtfeger R, Bondong A, Huber G, Kleindienst N, et al. Effects of a partly self-administered exercise program before, during, and after allogeneic stem cell transplantation. Blood 2011;117:2604-13.

[14] Bade BC, Thomas DD, Scott JB, Silvestri GA. Increasing physical activity and exercise in lung cancer: reviewing safety, benefits, and application. J Thorac Oncol 2015;10:861-71.

[15] Granger CL, McDonald CF, Berney S, Chao C, Denehy L. Exercise intervention to improve exercise capacity and health related quality of life for patients with Non-small cell lung cancer: a systematic review. Lung Cancer 2011;72:139-53.

[16] Sprod LK, Fernandez ID, Janelsins MC, Peppone LJ, Atkins JN, Giguere J, et al. Effects of yoga on cancer-related fatigue and global side-effect burden in older cancer survivors. J Geriatr Oncol 2015;6:8-14.

[17] Aydin T, Taspinar O, Kepekci M, Keskin Y, Erten B, Gunel M, et al. Functional independence measure scores of patients with hemiplegia followed up at home and in university hospitals. J Phys Ther Sci 2016;28(2):553- 7.

[18] Ng Y S, Astrid S, Silva D, Tan MLD, Tan YL, Chiew E. Functional outcomes after inpatient rehabilitation in a prospective stroke cohort. Proceed Singapore Healthcare 2013;22(3):175-82.

[19] Cheville AL, Troxel AB, Basford JR, Kornblith AB. Prevalence and treatment patterns of physical impairments in patients with metastatic breast cancer. J Clin Oncol 2008;26: 2621-9.

[20] Stubblefield MD, Schmitz KH, Ness KK. Physical functioning and rehabilitation for the cancer survivor. Semin Oncol 2013;40:784- 95.

[21] Smith A, Crouch S, Lax S, Li J, Painter D, Howell D, et al. Lymphoma incidence, survival and prevalence 2004–2014: sub-type analyses from the UK's haematological malignancy research network. Br J Cancer 2015;112:1575-84.

[22] Morton LM, Wang SS, Devesa SS, Hartge P, Weisenburger DD, Linet MS. Lymphoma incidence patterns by WHO subtype in the United States, 1992-2001. Blood 2006;107:265-76.

[23] Denlinger CS, deShazo M, Extermann M, et al. Senior adult oncology. J Natl Compr Canc Netw 2012;10 (2):162-209.

[24] Fu MR, Axelrod D, Guth A A, Cleland CM, Ryan CE, Weaver KR, et al. Comorbidities and quality of life among breast cancer survivors: A prospective study. J Pers Med 2015;26:5(3):229-42.

[25] Ahles TA, Saykin AJ. Breast cancer chemotherapy-related cognitive dysfunction. Clin Breast Cancer 2002;3(Suppl 3):S84-90.

[26] Jim HS, Phillips KM, Chait S, Faul LA, Popa MA, Lee YH, et al. Meta-analysis of cognitive functioning in breast cancer survivors previously treated with standard-dose chemotherapy. J Clin Oncol 2012;30:3578-87.

[27] Rodin G, Ahles TA. Accumulating evidence for the effect of chemotherapy on cognition. J Clin Oncol 2012;30:3568-9.

[28] Salbach NM, O'Brien K, Brooks D, Irvin E, Martino R, Takhar P, et al. Speed and distance requirements for community ambulation: a systematic review. Arch Phys Med Rehabil 2014;95:117-28.

[29] Cherrier MM, Anderson K, David D, Higano C, Gray H, Church A, et al. A randomized trial of cognitive rehabilitation in cancer survivors: A preliminary study. Life Sci 2013;93(17). Doi: 10.1016/j.lfs.2013.08.011.

[30] Mustian KM, Sprod LK, Janelsins M, Peppone LJ, Mohile S. Exercise recommendations for cancer-related fatigue, cognitive impairment, sleep problems, depression, pain, anxiety, and physical dysfunction: A Review. Oncol Hematol Rev 2012;8(2):81-8.

In: Clinical Oncology
Editors: Ariel Tenenbaum et al.
ISBN: 978-1-53617-933-0

Chapter 16

WOULD PHYSICAL ACTIVITY IMPROVE QUALITY OF LIFE IN PATIENTS WITH ADVANCED CANCER?

Gina Wong*[1]*, Emily Lam*[1]*,
Leah Drost*[1]*, Caitlin Yee*[1]*,
Edward Chow*[1,*]*, Ariel Tenenbaum*[2-4]*, MD
and Joav Merrick*[3-6]*, MD, MMedSci, DMSc
[1]Sunnybrook Health Sciences Centre, University of Toronto, Toronto, Ontario, Canada
[2]Center for Children with Chronic Diseases and Down Syndrome Center, Jerusalem, Israel
[3]Department of Pediatrics, Mt Scopus Campus, Hadassah Hebrew University Medical Center, Jerusalem, Israel
[4]National Institute of Child Health and Human Development, Jerusalem, Israel
[5]Kentucky Children's Hospital, University of Kentucky, Lexington, Kentucky, United States of America

[*] Corresponding Author's Email: Edward.Chow@sunnybrook.ca.

[6]Center for Healthy Development, School of Public Health, Georgia State University, Atlanta, Georgia, United States of America

ABSTRACT

Palliative cancer patients often experience more chronic pain, fatigue and depression than patients undergoing adjuvant treatment, leading to an overall reduction in quality of life. Patients with pain and fatigue tend to be more inactive, as they do not want to increase their pain. Sedentary behaviour can cause muscle atrophy and decreased bone density, leading to more pain and decreased mobility. Within the general population, physical activity is known to have multiple benefits such as stress relief, increased energy levels, reduction in cardiovascular disease risk and pain reduction. Therefore, we suggest to also use this treatment for people with cancer.

INTRODUCTION

Palliative cancer patients often experience more chronic pain, fatigue and depression than patients undergoing adjuvant treatment, leading to an overall reduction in quality of life (QoL) (1). Patients who have pain and fatigue tend to be more inactive, as they do not want to increase their pain (2). Sedentary behaviours can cause muscle atrophy and decreased bone density, leading to more pain and decreased mobility (3). Within the general population, physical activity (PA) is known to have multiple benefits such as stress relief, increased energy levels, reduction in cardiovascular disease risk and pain reduction (4, 5). A systematic review of physical activity in advanced cancer patients with bone metastases reported that even in fragile patients, supervised and individualized light PA was beneficial. In a single arm study of advanced male cancer patients, 30 minutes of supervised resistance and aerobic training twice a week for six weeks, followed by once a week for another 6 weeks improved fatigue scores at six months follow-up ($p = 0.007$); there were no adverse effects or increased risk of fractures caused by PA (6). Similarly another study allocated advanced cancer patients to either a 12-day PA or control group and compared Edmonton symptom assessment (ESAS) scores before and after the intervention; fatigue and drowsiness were significantly improved in the PA group, ($p < 0.01$ and $p < 0.05$, respectively) (7). These studies demonstrate a positive association between PA levels and improved health and well-being.

A recent study by Wallston et al. (8) showed that 88% of terminal cancer patients wished they were more mobile. Many patients were afraid to be physically active, and this sedentary behaviour likely contributed to their anxiety and poor mobility and functional status, thus reducing QoL (2,9). A qualitative study by Cheville et al. (2) identified common themes in patients' attitudes towards PA: most patients felt treatment was increasing their fatigue and regular daily activities were becoming increasingly difficult, but most also noticed that remaining active and doing familiar activities helped boost their wellbeing. (2). Based on the known benefits of PA, supervised PA can help maintain muscle mass and strengthen bones, allowing patients to improve balance and confidence in their physical functioning. PA programs can also help patients feel less defined by their illness and be able to do fairly normal activities rather than remaining bedridden. PA programs can therefore alleviate some of the physical and psychological factors that negatively impact QoL in patients with advanced cancer.

Although there have been multiple levels of evidence on the efficacy of PA in improving palliative cancer patients' QoL, healthcare professionals often overlook simple, inexpensive lifestyle changes like PA and often turn to invasive medical pain management treatments. Healthcare professionals should be encouraged to prescribe mild to moderate PA to complement other pain medications. Hopefully, increased emphasis on PA programs and more referrals from healthcare providers will encourage hospital-run PA programs as a standard component of palliative care. This could be a cost-effective way to decrease pain and increase QoL with a low risk of complications.

THIS BOOK

In this book we have gathered recent research related to cancer and cancer treatment and care. We believe that healthcare professionals should be encouraged to prescribe mild to moderate physical activity to complement other pain medications for people with cancer in palliative care. We also present research on pharmacy in cancer treatment, breast cancer, bone metastases, radiation therapy, pilot programs on telemedicine in cancer care, prostate cancer screening in Guyana, cost analysis of metastatic non-small cell lung cancer in Canada and early oncology rehabilitation for lymphoma patients in Singapore. We hope this research will be of interest to our readers.

ACKNOWLEDGMENTS

We thank the generous support of Bratty Family Fund, Michael and Karyn Goldstein Cancer Research Fund, Joey and Mary Furfari Cancer Research Fund, Pulenzas Cancer Research Fund, Joseph and Silvana Melara Cancer Research Fund, and Ofelia Cancer Research Fund.

REFERENCES

[1] Sandgren A, Fridlund B, Nyberg P, Strang P, Petersson K, Thulesius H. Symptoms, care needs and diagnosis in palliative cancer patients in acute care hospitals: A 5-year follow-up survey. Acta Oncol (Madr) 2010;49(4):460–6.

[2] Cheville AL, Dose AM, Basford JR, Rhudy LM. Insights into the reluctance of patients with late-stage cancer to adopt exercise as a means to reduce their symptoms and improve their function. J Pain Symptom Manage 2012;44(1):84–94.

[3] Berg HE, Eiken O, Miklavcic L, Mekjavic IB. Hip, thigh and calf muscle atrophy and bone loss after 5-week bedrest inactivity. Eur J Appl Physiol 2007;99(3):283–9.

[4] Keogh JWL, MacLeod RD. Body composition, physical fitness, functional performance, quality of life, and fatigue benefits of exercise for prostate cancer patients: A systematic review. J Pain Symptom Manage 2012;43(1):96–110.

[5] De Moor MHM, Beem AL, Stubbe JH, Boomsma DI, De Geus EJC. Regular exercise, anxiety, depression and personality: A population-based study. Prev Med (Baltim) 2006;42(4):273–9.

[6] Sheill G, Guinan EM, Peat N, Hussey J. Considerations for exercise prescription in patients with bone Mmetastases: A comprehensive narrative review. PM R 2018;10(8):843–64.

[7] Pyszora A, Budzyński J, Wójcik A, Prokop A, Krajnik M. Physiotherapy programme reduces fatigue in patients with advanced cancer receiving palliative care: randomized controlled trial. Support Care Cancer 2017;25(9):2899–908.

[8] Wallston KA, Burger C, Smith RA, Baugher RJ. Comparing the quality of death for hospice and non-hospice cancer patients. Med Care 1988;26(2):177–82.

[9] Dahele M, Skipworth RJE, Wall L, Voss A, Preston T, Fearon KCH. Objective physical activity and self-reported quality of life in patients receiving palliative chemotherapy. J Pain Symptom Manage 2007;33(6):676–85.

SECTION SIX: ACKNOWLEDGMENTS

In: Clinical Oncology
Editors: Ariel Tenenbaum et al.
ISBN: 978-1-53617-933-0

Chapter 17

About the Editors

Ariel Tenenbaum, MD is the director of the Center for Children with Chronic Diseases at the Hadassah-Hebrew University Medical Center at the Mount Scopus Campus, Jerusalem, Israel. He graduated the Hadassah-Hebrew University Medical School and after pediatric residency at the Department of Pediatrics at Mount Scopus Campus, he continued his work at the hospital as a senior pediatric consultant and teacher of medical students. In 2004 he was appointed the head of the new Israeli Down syndrome program in the hospital. In 2005 he started the pre-adoption clinic together with Professor Isaiah D. Wexler. In 2012 he opened the Hadassah Intellectual and Developmental Disability Multidisciplinary Evaluation Center in collaboration with the Ministry of Social Affairs. He co-founded the Disability Studies Center at the Hebrew University, where he teaches students from humanities and social studies. He was recently appointed as a child development consultant. In 2019 he was elected to the Israeli Pediatric Association Committee and serves as its scientific secretary. His main research topics are disabilities, adoption, chronic diseases and general pediatrics. He has published numerous book chapters, edited several books, and published dozens of scientific articles in international journals. E-mail: tene@hadassah.org.il

Victoria Rico, BSc(C) is an undergraduate student who is currently enrolled in the Honours Health Studies Program in the faculty of Applied Health Sciences at the University of Waterloo in Ontario, Canada. Currently working towards the completion of a Bachelor of Science, she is also enrolled in the co-operative education program at the University of Waterloo, through which she has completed work terms at the Sunnybrook Odette Cancer Centre (OCC) in Toronto, Ontario. Working as a clinical research assistant at the OCC, Victoria has led several research projects, including a retrospective review on a pharmacy callback program, a cross-sectional study examining the oral anti-cancer medication counselling program at the OCC, and three literature reviews on oncology-related topics. She presented her research findings from the pharmacy callback program at the Multinational Association of Supportive Care in Cancer conference in June 2019, and at the Canadian Association of Pharmacy in Oncology in April 2019. Further, she has co-authored on multiple scientific articles published in scholarly journals, and was a reviewer for The Breast Journal. E-mail: victoria.g.rico@hotmail.com

Carlo DeAngelis, PharmD is an oncology pharmacist and clinician scientist at the Odette Cancer Centre, Sunnybrook Health Sciences Centre in Toronto, Canada. He graduated from the University of Toronto with a Bachelor of Science in Pharmacy and subsequently earned his Doctor of Pharmacy from the State University of New York at Buffalo. Presently, Carlo is the Clincian Scientist for Oncology at the Odette Cancer Centre and owns and manages a community pharmacy in Woodbridge, Ontario. Further, he leads the Cannabis Consultation Service at the Odette Cancer Centre, which serves to guide patients with cancer on the use of cannabis. He is also an Associate Professor at the Leslie Dan Faculty of Pharmacy at University of Toronto where he lectures both Undergraduate Bachelor of Science in Pharmacy and Doctor of Pharmacy programs. Carlo has led many research projects, and has published several articles in the field of oncology. Through his contributions, Carlo has become a recognized leader in the field of oncology and in understanding side-effects associated with cancer treatment. Carlo's research mainly focuses on the immune system's involvement in contributing to side-effects of anti-cancer therapies. In 2011, Carlo was the president for the Canadian Association of Pharmacy in Oncology and in 2016, Carlo was named the Pharmacist of the Year by the Ontario Pharmacists Association. E-mail: carlo.deangelis @sunnybrook.ca

Joav Merrick, MD, MMedSci, DMSc, born and educated in Denmark is professor of pediatrics, Division of Pediatrics, Hadassah Hebrew University Medical Center, Mt Scopus Campus, Jerusalem, Israel and Kentucky Children's Hospital, University of Kentucky, Lexington, Kentucky United States and professor of public health at the Center for Healthy Development, School of Public Health, Georgia State University, Atlanta, United States, the former medical director of the Health Services, Division for Intellectual and Developmental Disabilities, Ministry of Social Affairs and Social Services, Jerusalem, the founder and director of the National Institute of Child Health and Human Development in Israel. Numerous publications in the field of pediatrics, child health and human development, rehabilitation, intellectual disability, disability, health, welfare, abuse, advocacy, quality of life and prevention. Received the Peter Sabroe Child Award for outstanding work on behalf of Danish Children in 1985 and the International LEGO-Prize ("The Children's Nobel Prize") for an extraordinary contribution towards improvement in child welfare and well-being in 1987. In 2017 appointed a Kentucky Colonel by the Commonwealth of Kentucky, the highest honor the governor can bestow to a person. E-mail: jmerrick@zahav.net.il

In: Clinical Oncology
Editors: Ariel Tenenbaum et al.
ISBN: 978-1-53617-933-0

Chapter 18

About the Center for Children with Chronic Diseases and Down Syndrome Center Jerusalem, Israel, Department of Pediatrics, Mt Scopus Campus, Hadassah Hebrew University Medical Center, Jerusalem, Israel

Chronic illnesses are common among children. These conditions last longer than a year and require continuous medical care and special needs. It is estimated that 10-20% of children in developed countries have one or more chronic condition. Advances in medicine and technology lead to an increase in the survival rate and longevity of children with chronic diseases and special needs. The severity of different chronic illnesses is variable, but there are many similarities. The child with a chronic illness faces physical, social, and emotional challenges. Therefore, medical care is not sufficient without rehabilitative service and emotional care for the child and his family.

Chronic illnesses are time and energy consuming. These children go through treatments, procedures and many healthcare visits. At home they often continue treatments as well, e.g., physiotherapy, breathing support machines and medications. This lifestyle may have detrimental effect on the child's social and emotional well-being, and similarly affect his parents and siblings.

CENTER FOR CHILDREN WITH CHRONIC DISEASES

The aim of the Center for Children with Chronic Diseases at the Hadassah-Hebrew University Medical Center at the Mount Scopus Campus, Jerusalem, is to enhance medical care, comfort and well-being of patients and their families in the hospital and beyond. The center provides integrated and comprehensive care for these patients. This includes extensive support services and helping their families cope with the burden of care.

Numerous pediatric specialty programs and medical divisions have been established in the center to care for specific chronic conditions; among them are cystic fibrosis, Down syndrome, diabetes mellitus, familial dysautonomia, neuromuscular diseases, rheumatic diseases, feeding disorders and metabolic diseases. All these programs include evaluation and support from common services in the center: Nursing, nutrition, psycho-social care, speech therapy, physiotherapy and more.

The center works as a "one stop shop" for these children; As many services as possible, under one roof, on the same visit. Centralizing the care enables parents to come to one location to receive care. The physicians and nurses coordinate the care of the children thereby alleviating some of the burden of care off the families.

Children who are included in the programs of the center usually need returning visits to various medical specialists, consultations by multidisciplinary health professionals and performing diagnostic tests e.g., blood work, x-rays and respiratory functions. Some children may need hospitalization or palliative care. The center can concentrate all diagnostic and follow-up testing, medical surveillance and treatment in the hands of an experienced staff who knows the child and his unique situation.

The center is situated close to the entrance of the hospital and the families can access it without going through the main hospital building. In the center there are ten rooms for consultations. In addition, there are dedicated rooms for tests, e.g., respiratory functions, blood tests, sweat test and more. There is a large space with eight beds for continuous treatments, for example intravenous immunoglobulins and biological medications. In this space several unique tests are performed as well, for example growth hormone test and allergy challenge tests. There is also a special room for procedures, in which children can go through painful treatments with appropriate anesthetics and surveillance.

A special classroom in the center is operated by the ministry of education. In the classroom, children can continue their studies or play and interact with other children, in arts and crafts and many other programs.

The center is surrounded by a large healing garden that is partially maintained by the children themselves.

CONCLUSION

In conclusion, we believe that the "all inclusive" model of a center for children with chronic conditions is beneficial for the children and their families in terms of health and quality of life, and that this model is currently the best service for them.

CONTACT

Ariel Tenenbaum, MD, Isaiah D Wexler, MD, PhD
Center for Children with Chronic Diseases, Department of Pediatrics, Mt Scopus Campus, Hadassah Hebrew University Medical Center, Jerusalem, Israel
E-mail: TENE@hadassah.org.il

In: Clinical Oncology ISBN: 978-1-53617-933-0
Editors: Ariel Tenenbaum et al.

Chapter 19

About the National Institute of Child Health and Human Development in Israel

The National Institute of Child Health and Human Development (NICHD) in Israel was established in 1998 as a virtual institute under the auspices of the Medical Director, Ministry of Social Affairs and Social Services in order to function as the research arm for the Office of the Medical Director. In 1998 the National Council for Child Health and Pediatrics, Ministry of Health and in 1999 the Director General and Deputy Director General of the Ministry of Health endorsed the establishment of the NICHD.

Mission

The mission of a National Institute for Child Health and Human Development in Israel is to provide an academic focal point for the scholarly interdisciplinary study of child life, health, public health, welfare, disability, rehabilitation, intellectual disability and related aspects of human development. This mission includes research, teaching, clinical work, information and public service activities in the field of child health and human development.

Service and Academic Activities

Over the years many activities became focused in the south of Israel due to collaboration with various professionals at the Faculty of Health Sciences (FOHS) at the Ben Gurion University of the Negev (BGU). Since 2000 an affiliation with the Zusman Child Development Center at the Pediatric Division of Soroka University Medical Center has resulted in collaboration around the establishment of the Down Syndrome Clinic at that center. In 2002 a full course on "Disability" was established at the Recanati School for Allied Professions in the Community, FOHS, BGU and in 2005 collaboration was started with the Primary Care Unit of the faculty and disability became part of the master of public health course on "Children and society". In the academic year 2005-2006 a one semester course on "Aging with disability" was started as part of the master of science program in gerontology in our collaboration with the Center for Multidisciplinary Research in Aging. In 2010 collaborations with the Division of Pediatrics, Hadassah Hebrew University Medical Center, Jerusalem, Israel around the National Down Syndrome Center and teaching students and residents about intellectual and developmental disabilities as part of their training at this campus.

Research Activities

The affiliated staff have over the years published work from projects and research activities in this national and international collaboration. In the year 2000 the International Journal of Adolescent Medicine and Health and in 2005 the International Journal on Disability and Human Development of

De Gruyter Publishing House (Berlin and New York) were affiliated with the National Institute of Child Health and Human Development. From 2008 also the International Journal of Child Health and Human Development (Nova Science, New York), the International Journal of Child and Adolescent Health (Nova Science) and the Journal of Pain Management (Nova Science) affiliated and from 2009 the International Public Health Journal (Nova Science) and Journal of Alternative Medicine Research (Nova Science). All peer-reviewed international journals.

NATIONAL COLLABORATIONS

Nationally the NICHD works in collaboration with the Faculty of Health Sciences, Ben Gurion University of the Negev; Department of Physical Therapy, Sackler School of Medicine, Tel Aviv University; Autism Center, Assaf HaRofeh Medical Center; National Rett and PKU Centers at Chaim Sheba Medical Center, Tel HaShomer; Department of Physiotherapy, Haifa University; Department of Education, Bar Ilan University, Ramat Gan, Faculty of Social Sciences and Health Sciences; College of Judea and Samaria in Ariel and in 2011 affiliation with Center for Pediatric Chronic Diseases and National Center for Down Syndrome, Department of Pediatrics, Hadassah Hebrew University Medical Center, Mount Scopus Campus, Jerusalem.

INTERNATIONAL COLLABORATIONS

Internationally with the Department of Disability and Human Development, College of Applied Health Sciences, University of Illinois at Chicago; Strong Center for Developmental Disabilities, Golisano Children's Hospital at Strong, University of Rochester School of Medicine and Dentistry, New York; Centre on Intellectual Disabilities, University of Albany, New York; Centre for Chronic Disease Prevention and Control,

Health Canada, Ottawa; Chandler Medical Center and Children's Hospital, Kentucky Children's Hospital, Section of Adolescent Medicine, University of Kentucky, Lexington; Chronic Disease Prevention and Control Research Center, Baylor College of Medicine, Houston, Texas; Division of Neuroscience, Department of Psychiatry, Columbia University, New York; Institute for the Study of Disadvantage and Disability, Atlanta; Center for Autism and Related Disorders, Department Psychiatry, Children's Hospital Boston, Boston; Department of Pediatric and Adolescent Medicine, Western Michigan University Homer Stryker MD School of Medicine, Kalamazoo, Michigan, United States; Department of Paediatrics, Child Health and Adolescent Medicine, Children's Hospital at Westmead, Westmead, Australia; International Centre for the Study of Occupational and Mental Health, Düsseldorf, Germany; Centre for Advanced Studies in Nursing, Department of General Practice and Primary Care, University of Aberdeen, Aberdeen, United Kingdom; Quality of Life Research Center, Copenhagen, Denmark; Nordic School of Public Health, Gottenburg, Sweden, Scandinavian Institute of Quality of Working Life, Oslo, Norway; The Department of Applied Social Sciences (APSS) of The Hong Kong Polytechnic University Hong Kong.

TARGETS

Our focus is on research, international collaborations, clinical work, teaching and policy in health, disability and human development and to establish the NICHD as a permanent institute in Israel in order to conduct model research.

CONTACT

Professor Joav Merrick, MD, MMedSci, DMSc
National Institute of Child Health and Human Development,
Jerusalem, Israel.
E-mail: jmerrick@zahav.net.il

SECTION SEVEN: INDEX

INDEX

A

B

C

D

E

F

G

H